# SC

# RECIPES

The Ultimate Beginners Guide to Effectively Make
Natural Soaps at Home

(The Ultimate Guide Book for Beginners to Learn
Homemade Soap)

**Alice Holmes**

Published by Oliver Leish

**Alice Holmes**

All Rights Reserved

*Soap Making Recipes: The Ultimate Beginners Guide to Effectively Make Natural Soaps at Home (The Ultimate Guide Book for Beginners to Learn Homemade Soap)*

ISBN 978-1-77485-078-7

Legal & Disclaimer

The information contained in this book is not designed to replace or take the place of any form of medicine or professional medical advice. The information in this book has been provided for educational and entertainment purposes only.

The information contained in this book has been compiled from sources deemed reliable, and it is accurate to the best of the Author's knowledge; however, the Author cannot guarantee its accuracy and validity and cannot be held liable for any errors or omissions. Changes are periodically made to this book. You must consult your doctor or get professional medical advice before using any of the suggested remedies, techniques, or information in this book.

Upon using the information contained in this book, you agree to hold harmless the Author from and against any damages, costs, and expenses, including any legal fees potentially resulting from the application of any of the information provided by this guide. This disclaimer applies to any damages or injury caused by the use and application, whether directly or indirectly, of any advice or information presented, whether for breach of contract, tort, negligence, personal injury, criminal intent, or under any other cause of action.

You agree to accept all risks of using the information presented inside this book. You need to consult a professional medical practitioner in order to ensure you are both able and healthy enough to participate in this program.

# Table of Contents

# Introduction

Have you actually ever used soap before?

Most people have never used soap in their entire lives.

And I don't refer to third-world countries, poor people, or just people who refuse to use soaps and maintain their "natural odor"...I speak about normal people who shower every day, wash their hands, and condition their hair. Yes, that's right – that includes you.

Commercial soap sold in retail stores is mostly made from artificial chemicals, hardeners and synthetic lathering materials. Some of these ingredients are actually <u>dangerous</u> to your skin.

On the other hand, soaps that are made by the hand like they used to be made for centuries, are very beneficial to the skin and to your health and looks. Handmade soap is made from natural oils and liquids and does not contain harsh chemicals.

This book contains all the essential information about soap making:

What you need to get started

A step-by-step guide for different soap-making processes

And 100 simple soap recipes that every newbie can make.

The soap recipes in this book follow either the melt-and-pour method—for those who are not ready to deal with lye yet—or the cold process technique. Both are great for beginners and the instructions are explained in detail so you won't have to make any guesses or go back to the guide every time you make soap.

The recipes are grouped into three categories. In the first group, you will find recipes which require only four or five ingredients. Any one of them will be the perfect choice for your first ever handmade soap.

The second group is for beauty soaps, with each recipe indicating what it's best used for. They vary from simple four-ingredient melt-and-pour recipes to more complicated cold process soap recipes.

The last group of recipes is for making beautiful soaps with several colors, layers, or swirl patterns. Although these recipes are a bit challenging and take some practice to create, they're perfect for when you're ready to step up your soap-making game.

Lastly, you will learn how to use a lye calculator. While this isn't essential for beginners, knowing this may come in handy if you need to make small changes in the soap recipe.

# Chapter 1: All You Need To Know About Soap

Soaps, be it those tiny bars, sweet smelling hand soaps or the huge bars used for washing or cleaning clothes, soaps are a necessity in our lives. They keep us clean and we use them to maintain our hygiene, mostly. They are bought in bulk at the supermarket, local shop or online stores.

That bar of blue soap in your kitchen and the hand wash liquid soap in your washroom, maybe you read the ingredients and wondered what some of those things were and wondered how long it took to make them. Ingredients that go into soap are surprisingly very cheap, affordable and already in your kitchen, you just must know what you are adding and how and what else you require.

All soaps that we use require three basic ingredients: water, lye and mixing oils. They are the base of any soap that is out there in the market.

To get all scientific about soap, they are just acidic compounds that have been mixed together with a base to create a salt, which is soap. Sodium hydroxide, which in the manufacturing industry is referred to as lye is used to make bar soaps and potassium hydroxide is used to make liquid soaps. A blend of the two, carefully mixed together, the result will be a creamy soap that is the same consistency as thick pudding.

**History**

Once, in a land far far far away, Babylonians were making soap. This is after an excavation in ancient Babylon was done. According to the excavation, it is believed that the Babylonians were making soap in the era of 2800 B.C and they were the first people to master soap making. The soaps that they used were made from fats that were boiled with ashes. They used in the textile manufacturing industry, by cleaning cotton and wool and for, a very long period of 5000 years, it was used medicinally.

Not much has changed with how soap is being made in the current society we live and the previous, old past eras. The Egyptians were believed to be making soap by mixing vegetable and animal oils. this by the evidence provided by the Ebers papyrus (Egypt, 1550 B.C). The oils were then mixed with alkaline salts to get a soapy product.

In the first century A.D. Romans made soap from urine- yep, your excretion was soap once back in the day, hehe. The soap was something that many people knew of in the Roman Empire. Wood ashes and goat's tallow were the main ingredients of soap that Phoenicians used in 600BC.

Others like the Celts used plant ashes and animal fat to create soap. To them it was saipo, and the name we widely use today, soap, was derived from it. Meaning the Egyptians, Mesopotamian and ancient Romans and Greeks were the first people to use and make soap.

The soap that they made was not for cleaning their bodies like it is today, it was used to clean utensils, goods or as medicine.

Now to some facts about soap.

Soap, either as a bar or liquid, is made from natural ingredients of animal fats, plant products. These can be vegetable oils, such as coconut oil, olive oil.

The name "soap" is believed to have been linked to Mount Sapo in Rome, which is a belief that is quite popular, as "sapo" in

Latin translates to soap. The name was first noticed in Pliny the Elder's Historia Naturalis.

Finer soaps were introduced in the 16th Century in Europe as animal fats were swapped for vegetable oils like olive oil. In Europe, an example of such soaps still produced in the Castile soap that is made from Italy's oldest "white soap."

In the 18th century, soaps industrially made became popular. This was achieved when advertisements in America and Europe emphasized the importance of cleanliness to avoid being sick. Before the Industrial Revolution, soaps were made in small quantities and they were rough. In 1780 at Tipton, James Keir added chemical works so that sulfates from soda and potash were used to manufacture alkali. This was later added in the soap making industry.

In London, clear or transparent liquid soap was manufactured first in 1807 by Andrew Pears, with his son opening a factory later on in Isleworth in 1862. in America, Benjamin T. Babbitt, a manufacturer brought marketing innovations which had a bar of soap and samples of various products as well. The largest soap business Unilever came to be when brothers James and William Hesketh Lever in 1886 bought a soap works in Warrington and founded Lever Brothers before it was named Unilever. These large soap industries were the first to use advertisement campaigns in large scales.

In 1940, chemists uncovered that some naturally occurring substances' molecular structure could be altered, this resulted in detergent. It was a good discovery as detergent worked in both cold and/or hard water; with changes being made to make it suitable to clean out tough stains and dirt. Synthetic detergents or modern detergents have come a long way as they are now more sophisticated in so many ways.

Detergent now can be found in any form of cleaning products with soap being defined as anything that can clean and forms bubbles, more specifically if it is the form of a bar.

The most common process of making soap, in this century is the cold process. There is a hot process too, that is explained further in the book, but the cold process is how most soaps are made.

Making soap, does not require you to have a degree in Chemistry or have any knowledge of bases and acids, luckily or most of us would not even bother with it, I know I wouldn't have. The main thing to understand is that soap is made from blending vegetable oils or fats as well together with lye this acts as a solvent in the recipes. The molecules found in this bind together after constant knocking and bashing with each other to create soap through a process called saponification.

There are various soaps in the market, soaps nowadays have chemical fragrances, hardeners or lather boosters in their ingredients. It makes a whole lot of difference when it comes to which soap to purchase, as there are soaps that cost more than $5 while you can get a 3-pack for as little as $2.

With what we have researched and learned in the process of writing this book, and it is common knowledge, your skin is sensitive and all natural; therefore, why would you make your skin react due to what you expose it to? The recipes in here are all-natural products used and they work well with your skin. Dry skin is a result of chemical exposure to your skin for a long period of time.

Most soaps are made with lye; which can be deceptively hidden to you as the consumer by labeling it Sodium Tallowate, which is a mixture of lye (sodium hydroxide) and tallow (beef fat that has been rendered). it is a clever trick but manipulative in its own way.

The difference between you making your own product, which here is soap, and buying one from your favorite store and the one made eons ago is the vast array of high and better-quality ingredients that you, as the current reader of this book has been provided to you to make your soap better for your skin, smell unique and have all the right measurements for your ingredients. A vegan person can make their own soap without having to use animal fats, there are huge products to explore to get the soap to your liking.

In this book, we are going to learn how to make soap from animal fats, use lye and those you don't need to make using lye. To top it all off, you learn to make the soap that your skin will be okay with and the right substances in it and not just chemicals. It is easy to make soap, though there will be errors made, that is okay. Soap making is similar to cooking, you make mistakes before you become an expert. Let's look at the bases of soap, the ingredients you can use and additives that you can use.

Forward march!

# Chapter 2: 22 Best Handmade Soap Recipes For Bennere

Learn the Basics of Soapmaking

Before you get started, take a moment to familiarize yourself with the most common methods of soapmaking. Some of these processes are easier than others. Knowing how each one works will help you decide which tutorials you want to tackle.

Make sure to read all the instructions for each soap and take any necessary precautions. Some of these examples use lye, which can burn the skin and eyes if you're not careful.

Create Swirls of Color and Layer Multiple Fragrances

Cold process soap can be made by beginners, but only after learning about how to work with lye safely. Once you get

14

the basics down, coming up with different cold process soap recipes can be really rewarding. This example is eye-catching and smells heavenly

You'll Need:

Lye

Water

Coconut, canola, castor, and sesame oil

Shea and kokum butter

Lime, vetiver, and cedarwood essential oil

Kaolin clay

Activated charcoal

Cut Up Thin Orange Slices for a Citrusy Soap:

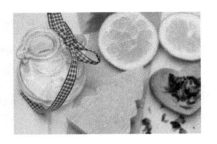

This soap recipe is simple because it uses a melt and pour base that is pre-mixed and ready to go. No need to work with messy chemicals! The citrus slices are something you'd only find in handmade soap.

You'll Need:

Goat's milk melt and pour base

Silicone soap molds

Citrus essential oil

Dried citrus slices

Exfoliate Your Skin With a Loofah Soap:

Loofah soaps are extremely easy to make when you purchase a melt and pour soap

16

base. All you need to do is melt the base and add any extras, cut the loofahs so they fit in the mold, then pour the soap on top of the loofah.

You'll Need:

Melt and pour base

Loofah

Rose essential oil

Rose mica

Soap mold

Make Soap Inspired by Your Favorite Tea:

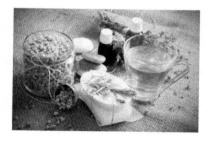

When making soap from scratch, try to find a simple soap recipe that utilizes oils you might already have in your kitchen. You can also examine your pantry for other ingredients that would work well in a bar of soap. In this case, green tea is used alongside eucalyptus and lemongrass essential oil.

You'll Need:

Palm oil and palm kernel oil

Coconut, olive, castor, soybean, and sunflower oil

Cocoa butter

Lye

Green tea

Steeped green tea leaves

Eucalyptus and lemongrass essential oil

The soap making equipment

For safely making homemade soap it is essential that the specific proportions of these soap ingredients are scrupulously followed.

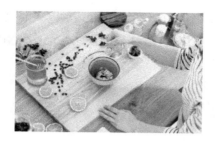

It is highly recommended that you use a specialised software to calculate the proportions for each ingredient and to run it every time a new recipe is tried. There are many types of softwares for this purpose. There are even iPhones apps.

Some basic equipment must be used when preparing soap ingredients and making soap:

- an accurate scale;

- an accurate quick reading thermometer;

- a few small measuring cups;a stick blender to blend the oils with the lye mixture and start the saponification process;

- and soap molds.

Here is an example of the proportions for the various soap ingredients:

- 450 grams of vegetable fat;

- 170 millilitres of water

- 60 grams of caustic soda

The soap making process

Preparation of soap ingredients

Soap making requires water, caustic alkali and fats or oils.

It is very important that caustic soda is gently poured into water, and NEVER the opposite which will cause a kind of explosion and splash corrosive product on your body. The temperature of the water and soda mixture naturally rises up to around 190°F, or 90°C.

Therefore a glass (Pyrex) or a stainless steel container is to be used. Do not use a plastic container as it would melt due to high temperature. Please remember that aluminium is corroded by soda. Always use wooden spoons to stir soda.

Mixing the soap ingredients

Soda temperature must lower down to 95-105°F (35-40°C) and oil must be heated up to 130°F (55°C). After checking those temperatures with an accurate quick reading thermometer, slowly pour caustic soda into the heated oil. As soon as the two ingredients are mixed, you can use a stick blender to blend the oil with the lye mixture. While stirring the lye-water-oil mixture with the stick blender, you turn on the blender in short bursts. Blend for 3 to 5 seconds and then stir some more.

Once you start using the stick blender, you may see the oil turn cloudy and the soap mixture begin to come together. Keep blending in short bursts until the oil and lye-water are completely mixed together. This should not take more than 30-40 seconds.

Now you are nearing the stage called "trace". Using the stick blender enables you to reach trace in under a minute whereas if you use a wooden or a plastic spoon it will take 10 to 75 minutes for the same result.

Successful soap making secret

Trace is the term to describe the consistency or thickness, and the stage where the handmade soap mixture is ready to be poured into molds. Tracing is easily recognized. Using a plastic spatula, drizzle a small amount across the top of the soap mixture. If a mark or trail remains for a few seconds before disappearing again, your soap has traced. The mixture should have the consistency of liquid honey or pudding.

Your personal touch in your homemade soap

It is now the right time for you to add your own additives (essential oils, honey, milk, etc) before pouring the mixture into the soap molds, which you would have lubricated already with vaseline.

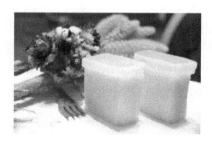

You may now cover the molds with a cloth and let them rest for 24 to 36 hours before getting hold of the soap. Indeed, saponification takes at least 24 hours to complete and, during this period, soap is still corrosive. You should be particularly careful to keep children away from it during this period of time.

After soap making

After this time, you can take the soaps off the molds, and rinse them to remove any excess of lye.

However, soaps are still rather soft, and you need to allocate around 6 weeks for them to be completely dry and hard.

Example of soap recipe:

Various soap recipes can be found on websites about soap. For example, here is a very simple recipe:

- 450 grams of coconut oil;

- 700 grams of olive oil;

- 450 grams of vegetable fat;

- 600 millilitres of water;

- 223 grams of caustic soda.

I could not believe it when my wife told me the supposed "natural" soap I was very happy to use was staining my shower screen; and it was true! She gave me a natural handmade soap, and it was a discovery for me. The peppermint soap was so sweet on my skin and so refreshing! I had never felt such a thing. This started my passion for natural handmade, homemade soaps. I begun searching what were soaps made of, and was terrified when I learned what they put in commercially-produced soaps! Straight away I decided I had the mission to inform people about the risks with soaps bought at the supermarket, and to promote natural homemade soaps. It was not a big deal for me as I was already a definite user of natural medicine with essential oils. I hope you'll enjoy reading and learning the techniques of bar or liquid soap making, and start making your own natural homemade soap!

Soap Isn't All Alike

A soapmaker recently asserted that all soap is basically the same, and there really is nothing proprietary to set one soap apart from another.

Excuse me! I don't think so.

There are dozens of ways to make soap that's different from the next person, not counting all the ways it differs from commercial products. She had her mind made up and, let's face it, some folks truly are not very creative.

## Chapter 3: Get Familiar With Soap Making Tools

Pretty much of what you are required to make a soap might already be in your house, kitchen in particular. You might have an old pan that you are not using anymore, some old spoons, plastic jugs, and whisks. Now, before throwing them out and start ordering unnecessary tools for making soap, take a look and find something that could be of use for making soap. After gathering what you found, then you can now start purchasing additional tools.

Keep in mind that you don't really need to get extravagant and spend a loads of bucks to get started with soap making, but of course you must have the basic tools in order to ensure that your soap will turn out great and that your friends and family are always safe if ever they decided try and use your soap. Remember that creating your soap will always be a chemistry, that's why you must always take it seriously as much as possible. Of course don't forget to have some fun!

Moulds

Obviously since it is moulds that we're talking about, it should come in all sizes and shapes, and different materials. As for me, my favourite kind of mould is a silicone because it is easy to pop the soap out and doesn't really need any prepping.

Of course, having some few plastic moulds can also be helpful if you are getting troubled of seeking a better mould but it's just that it is quite difficult to get your soap especially if you are not using any additional hardening ingredients.

A wooden box lined with wax paper is an example of soap moulds. For beginners, you might find this really helpful because a lot of individuals have a box around their house.

Moulds that are box will create a loaf of soap that you can just cut into pieces. In addition, woods will also help to insulate your soap so that your finished product won't have that much issue when you are on the stage of cooling your soap. Here's a great tip, if ever you had made a soap that looks opaque on the outside, and has a dark spot on the center, then the insulation during the soap making process was most likely the root.

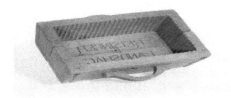

"A Wooden Mould"

Kitchen Scales

If you don't even have a digital kitchen scale, then I don't think you should think of attempting to make a natural soap. Don't worry because, this scale is not really expensive and is in fact quite easy to utilize.

Always remember that making soaps are exclusively in weight because attempting to measure in teaspoons or cups is very imprecise. Of course if we're talking about cakes and muffins this kind of measuring approach would be fine but not when you are making soap!

Digital kitchen scales works by measuring how much something weighs, and the point here is you must be consistent at all time. As for me, I am using some tiny volume types of measurements when I am adding some mineral pigments, but even if you end up with the same approach as I do, make sure that you also measure your dash, tad, smidgen, pinch, and a drop measuring spoons.

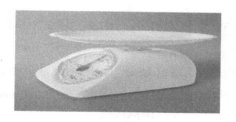

"Kitchen Scale"

Digital Thermometer

Since soap making does involve of melting, hardening, and curing, measuring temperature around your product is very crucial.

When mixing together your ingredients, you must ensure that the temperature is consistent from time to time, because if you don't do so, you might lose a batch. Of course, you can use standard thermometers if you don't have any digital ones, but the drawback is that using standard glass thermometers tend to get broken.

That's why it is highly suggested that you use an inexpensive digital kitchen thermometer because you can dip its tip to essential oils and your lye and water because of its stainless steel tip. On the other hand, if you are planning on utilizing glass thermometers, ensure that you get two in order to keep one submerged into melting oils, and one for a jug of lye-water.

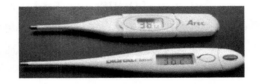

"Digital Thermometer"

Stick Blender

If you want to know the traditional approach of making natural soap, you must know that it actually involves standing over a pot and stirring for a long period of time. If you find it fun, then I don't encourage you not to try making soap this way.

It would practically help your lye-water and essential oils to chemically bond for about less than a couple of minutes. If you are planning on purchasing one, I highly suggest that you get a stick blender that has holes into it, so that you minimize the amount of air that will be taken into your soap to get rid of air bubbles as much as possible.

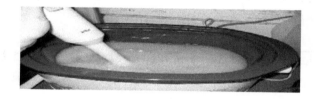

"Stick Blender"

Utensils

Let me get direct to the point. You must have different utensils for creating soap because as I've mentioned before, you will be dealing with chemical reactions.

☐ Get a stainless steel spoon for stirring essential oils. And a large one for stirring lye water.

☐ Get a stainless steel whisk to blend essential oils, botanicals, and minerals.

☐ Try also to get a stainless steel to pour your lye water and get strained. It would be a big help to get rid of lumps and un-dissolved lye, and also it is very helpful to eliminate possible air bubbles.

☐ And lastly, a silicone spatula would be really helpful to get as much soap out of your pan as possible.

Gloves and Goggles

Soap making is a fun and creative task. But if you are starting from scratch, then it is given that you will most likely handle sodium hydroxide aka lye. This extreme substance is really harmful if not treated accordingly.

But not unless you are planning on using the Melt and Pour method on which a large part of chemical process have already been done. As I've mentioned before, soap making is the process of chemical reaction between an alkali (i.e. lye) and an acid (i.e. essential oils). Long story short, after finishing the process of making soap, there will be no lye residue in your bars. Just always remember that when you are handling lye, you should be wearing a pair of gloves and a goggle. It would also be better if you wear a long sleeved shirt, and an apron.

And lastly, another safety gear that you might want to consider is a face mask because lye water can give off harmful vapours and who would be sane enough to inhale those in?

Remember that once you got splashed by a lye water mixture, you must immediately rinse the affected area to prevent further issues.

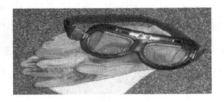

"Gloves and Googles For Handling Lye and Chemical Reactions"

Containers

Since soap making involves various kinds of essential oils and ingredients, it is always better to keep them in distance.

When picking a container, make sure that they are heat-proof, and if you pick any metal containers, ensure that they are stainless steel because some kind of metals will react with lye.

After using a particular container, don't ever use them for other use. It's for the sole purpose of soap making only!

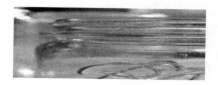

# Chapter 4: The Making Of Coconut

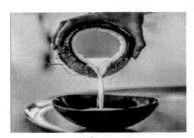

**Oil Soap**

Step 1: prepare the pink kaolin clay, use about 1.5 tablespoons of pink kaolin clay, add in one tablespoon of distilled water, and stir properly.

Step 2: measure the coconut oil; because coconut oil soap is very cleansing and can make the skin feel dry, it's advisable to use a 20% super fat to help counter that, melt the fat, then add the coconut oil and lye at about 78 degrees Fahrenheit.

Step 3: use your mixer to stir properly; when it's finally smoothed out and reached trace, pour into a cup and put in the hydrated pink clay, one teaspoon per cup of soap, blend very well with your mixer and pour into your mold, allow to cool. Your coconut oil soap is ready.

How to Make Aloe Vera Soap

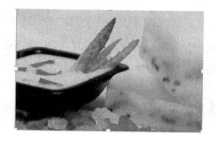

Step 1

First, you will be needing a soap base, aloe vera gel, or aloe vera body wash. So you will need to melt the soap base.

Step 2

Okay, so now that you have everything melted, your next step is to add the aloe vera gel or body wash, add a couple of pumps. Add a little bit of chopped up aloe vera. And then mix up.

Step 3

(This is completely optional) you are going to add some mica powder, which is green in color. And then some green soap coloring. You can do this if you want as it is optional. Now, you have your soap, so you are going to put them into your molds.

Mango and Coconut Milk Soap

Step 1

Get your fresh mango, peel off the back, and chop it into small pieces, then you blend it with a blender.

Step 2

Make use of a sieve to sieve it, to separate the chaff from the juice.

## Step 3

Get your olive oil, coconut oil, shea butter, and castor oil. Pour everything together including your fresh mango puree, pour in your coconut milk, and use your mixer to mix very well. Pour in your sodium hydroxide, mix properly, pour in your fragrance, and start pouring the mixture into your mold.

# Chapter 5: Types Of Soap

There are so many types of soap that are available in the market that it is sometimes hard to pick the right one for yourself. Now, the soaps are all alike which means that the action of soaps is the same. However, the ingredients that are used in the soap make all the difference.

It is not just a "psychological" thing to feel clean after a soapy bath, it is the ingredients used in soap that make them so effective in cleaning our body and also other surfaces that they are used at.

Soap is a cleaning product made from natural ingredients.

These ingredients may include both plant and animal products, including such items as:

- animal fat, such as tallow or vegetable oil, such as castor, olive, or coconut oil.
- plants such as soapwort or Western soapberry (aptly named!).
- rainwater.
- fragrances such as cinnamon, rose water, oil of bergamot or cloves.

Detergent, on the other hand, is a synthetic product. It often has petroleum-based ingredients, although there are plant-based detergents available as well.

One way of looking at types of soap is by origin. There are handmade and commercially made soaps. Another way to look at soap is by its use. Soap is available for personal use, laundry use, and dishwashing, and pet cleaning products that are soaps can also be found.

Kitchen soaps:

There are two common types of Kitchen soaps: cleansers and detergents.

Cleansers:

Cleansers are often made withand they are formulated to eliminate heavy oil or solid particles and hard-to-remove stains. The cleansers come in many different types depending on the type of abrasives they contain.

Detergents:

are made to remove tough grease and release the solid dirt particles in the foam that is produced by the detergent. There are two types of dish detergents:and .

**Transparent soaps:** Are soaps that feels good, lathers beautifully and leaves your skin feeling squeaky clean while not drying it. How does it do all this? Because the soap crystals in transparent soap are small and there is no unnecessary excess oil, the soap is, in effect, pre-dissolved and ready for action, and feels extremely smooth to the skin. It takes little effort to lather up thick, creamy lather, and it takes little effort to rinse. No residue is left on your skin or in the sink and tub. No residue means less clogged pores and blemishes and no soap scum to scrub clean.

Transparent soap has a long history dating back to 1789, when Andrew Pears first manufactured the bar that bears his name. Making soap transparent is an extra step for the soap maker, but one that is most worthwhile. Transparent soap can be made from palm and coconut oil as opaque soap, but usually the only liquid oil that is ever used is castor oil.

Soap is transparent when it contains no large crystals, and theoretically all opaque soap can be made transparent, although some oil combinations do not result in a very clear soap. Recipes for transparent soap are usually a closely guarded secret because of the amount of experimentation involved in achieving the desired results. If you've ever tried to make any soap yourself, you'll realize that the combinations of oil and the proportions of them are infinite.

Glycerine soaps:

Are simply soaps that have glycerine added to them, making them look somewhat translucent. Sometimes natural soap makers will refer to their opaque soaps as glycerine soaps as well just because they contain glycerine. All soap when made with fats and lye contain glycerine because it is a natural by-product of the saponification reaction. Mass-produced soap has the glycerine removed from the soap because it is worth more money to sell it separately than to leave it in the soap where it may benefit the skin. The large amount of extra glycerine in glycerine soaps causes the soap to absorb water from the humidity in your bathroom. Thi is the same reason these bars are so gentle: a small film of glycerine left on the skin draws moisture from the iar to your skin. All our soap can be used right down to the very last tiny sliver.

Novelty soaps:

Include the soap in the shape of a rubber ducky, made not only to clean, but for enjoyment as well. Soaps may be made novel by their shape and or coloring. There are novelty soaps for children. As with other types of soap, you can purchase novelty soaps or make your own. Many specialty soap molds are available in a vast array of ethnic, holiday, and other shapes.

Beauty soaps:

Are likely to feature attractive fragrances, and ingredients to address a variety of skin types. Beauty soaps may feature glycerin, or special oil blends.

Guest soaps:

Are usually miniature soaps, molded into attractive shapes and designed for use by guests in the main bathroom, or in a separate guest bathroom. Popular shapes are flowers, sea shells, and rounds.

Laundry soaps:

Are soaps specially formulated to clean clothes. Be sure to follow package directions for best results.

Personal soaps:

This kind of soap is made in many forms and special formulations for specific personal hygiene needs. One type of the personal soap isthat is made to prevent bacteria and viruses from spreading. There are also that have a mix of ingredients that cleans both the skin and hair.

Perfumed soaps:

Are produced by adding a fewand.

Guest soaps:

Arethat are made and shaped into attractive shapes and they are basically designed for the either in the main bathroom or separate guest bathroom. Popular and commonly used shapes are flowers, sea shells and rounds

Medicated soaps:

Are very similar to original soap. Unlike original soap, medicated soap has the .

Dish soaps:

Are the counterparts of dish detergent and are coming in a variety of scents. As with laundry soap, be sure to follow package directions, and do not use dish soap in a dishwasher.

# Chapter 6: Be Prepared!

Safety is a central element in the successful manufacture of soap. Working with sodium hydroxide means you must be attentive and committed to what you are doing. Rubber gloves and even safety goggles are a good addition to your fundamental arrangements.

Due to the tendency of soap to adhere to surfaces until it is thoroughly washed off, you will need separate bowls and utensils especially for your soap-making. Glass jars and bowls are always good when handling oils as there is no transfer, seeping or filtering into the container, as may be possible with plastic.

Pay attention to the fact that lye will react with aluminum so when heating it, ensure that you never use aluminum pans. Non-stick and stainless steel pans work best.

Your work surface needs to be able to withstand the very hot temperatures so make sure that it is suitable – granite, marble – or make sure you protect it with suitable coverings, cloths and even newspaper. Newspaper is handy because it can be discarded after use. Old newspaper can be composted and only any stained paper, from spills, needs find its way into the dustbin.

You will need a thermometer to gauge the temperature, a few rubber spatulas, molds which can be anything simple, even old margarine tubs or yoghurt cartons. You can also use a lined cake pan- as a mold – lined with cling wrap or wax paper. You also need a kitchen scale, paper towels or kitchen roll, at least 2 bowls (for the oils) and an immersion blender which is just something to stir with and 2 glass jars for the lye and the water.

So the list needs to include:

Rubber gloves, safety goggles, several separate containers, bowls and utensils especially for the soap-making, non-stick or stainless steel pots and pans, a large double-boiler, a suitable work surface, newspaper, a thermometer, rubber spatulas, molds (margarine tubs, yoghurt cartons, cake molds), a kitchen scale, an immersion blender or stirrer and at least 2 glass jars.

# Chapter 7: 20 Tips To Make Every Homemade Soap Bar Amazing

As a beginner, expect that there will be challenges along the way. But what's great about the soap making process is that your efforts are never in vain. Your failures, no matter how bad you think they are, can become opportunities to learn so much more. Once you get used to the process, and you start to pick up your own tricks along the way, your soap making possibilities are limitless. Here are a few tips that I would like to share with you that will help you make every homemade soap bar amazing.

Measure all your ingredients are already prepared before you get started. Time is of the essence when making your own soap. You need to act fast and have an organized work flow. Measuring your ingredients ahead of time not only makes your work much easier, but it also gives you the chance to do a quick check if there are any ingredients you might have missed.

Always use a lye calculator when planning your soap recipes. If you're unsure of how much lye to use in your lye-based soap recipes, you can always use a lye calculator online. This takes out the guesswork of figuring out the right lye-oil ratio and you get a better chance of making a solid soap.

Use silicone molds. While there's nothing wrong with using all sorts of materials as molds, silicone molds are your best bet if you're aiming for a consistent shape. Silicone molds make soap removable a breeze and there's less chances of chipping the soap. Simply tap the soap out when it's hardened and you're all done.

Do a supplies inventory regularly. There's nothing worse than getting a spark of soap inspiration and quickly finding out that you don't have enough supplies to turn your ideas into reality. Even if you say you're just a beginner at this point, having a good supply of the common soap making ingredients is a great way to motivate yourself to get better at your craft.

Get great deals on ingredients by buying bulk or checking the sale aisles. Once you've tasted success in your first batch of homemade soap, it's really hard to fight the urge to make more. You'll end up making more soap anyway so you might as well get your money's worth now by looking for great deals on ingredients.

Mix dried herbs with vitamin E oil to preserve its color. While it's just natural for dried herbs to turn brown once it starts to oxidize, you can slow the process by mixing the herbs with some vitamin E oil.

Add a few drops of sunflower oil to melt and pour soap if you want to get a boost of nutrients. Sunflower oil is one of the most versatile beauty oils in the world and is known for its endless list of benefits.

Warm up cold honey before adding it to the soap mixture. Cold honey has the tendency to congeal and clump. Make sure to warm it up in the microwave in advance to get a smooth soap mixture.

When in doubt, less is more. Take the soap making process one step at a time so that there's less chances of making mistakes. For example, when heating the soap base in the microwave, try to use short bursts. This way, you won't end up with a big mess because the soap base boiled over from too much heat. You should also use scents sparingly, adding more if you want to get a stronger scent. The same goes for colorants. Try not to overload your homemade soap with pigment as it can cause skin staining if you use too much.

Clear your sense of smell with coffee grounds. It's easy to overload your sense of smell when you're working with many essential oils at once. So before you check the scent of a soap batch one last time, make sure to sniff some coffee grounds. This way, you'll have a true sense of the scent and you can add more if you think it's too faint.

Mix powdered ingredients with oil for a smoother finish. This way, there's a lesser chance of the powdered ingredients clumping when added to the soap base. Using water to dilute powdered ingredients could make the soap mixture lumpy.

Keep vinegar close for quick lye clean ups. No matter how careful you try to be, you can't avoid getting a few beads of lye on your workspace, or worse, yourself! Vinegar is the best way to neutralize the lye so you don't end up with a messy problem. Soak little rags in vinegar before you start working so you can quickly grab one when you need it.

Cover new soap with plastic wrap to prevent soda ash. Soda ash can make soap look sloppy and dirty so to prevent it from forming, make sure to put plastic wrap on top of new soap before setting it aside for curing. While soda ash is completely harmless, it could ruin the aesthetic value of your artisanal soap.

Prevent bubbles with a spritz of isopropyl alcohol. Another common problem that first time soap makers encounter is the formation of bubbles on top of the soap. Just like soda ash, this can affect your soap's aesthetic value. One way to prevent bubble from forming is to lightly spritz the top of soap with alcohol after pouring the soap base into the mold. This should be enough to take care of those bubbles.

Have a dedicated cutting board for your soap creations. This way, you won't risk contaminating your food with soap particles from your last DIY project. Don't forget to draw lines on your cutting board so that you have guidelines for cutting your soap. Now you don't have to guess if you cut your soap bars straight.

Wait at least 3 days before cleaning your soap making equipment if you worked with lye. It may sound counterintuitive but cleaning your soap equipment right away will only leave you with a greasy mess. Also, it will expose you to raw lye, which could lead to allergic reactions and irritation. Waiting it out for a few days will eventually turn the lye and soap grease into soap that you'll be able to easily rinse off. Just soak in hot water and you'll be done with clean up.

Donate surplus soap to your local homeless shelter. Once you get into the craze of making homemade soap, it's just a matter of months before you realize that you have enough soap to clean an entire village with. Instead of letting surplus and imperfect soap go to waste, donate it to your local homeless shelter. There many non-profits out there who are always in need of personal care items. This is your chance to be a blessing and share a simple, but meaningful gift to the less fortunate.

Get creative with your soap creations. The great thing about soap making is that you are only limited by your creativity. You can make soap with just about anything so you can customize your soap according to your preference and skin needs.

Practice makes perfect. While we're all familiar with this saying, this is especially true in soap making. Expect to make mistakes along the way, especially when you're working with lye. Don't get discouraged when your first batch doesn't turn out the way you want it. As long as you know at what point you might have gotten it wrong, you always have another chance to get it right on your next try.

Even the best soap makers had to learn from their mistakes.

Don't forget to have fun. Soap making is not just about creating the perfect bar. It's also about creating something beautiful out of a few basic ingredients. While there's nothing wrong with striving for perfection, focusing too much on the end product might cause you to miss out on other fun aspects of soap making, like experimenting with essential oils to get your signature scent or working with your family to create the best bath soap for all of you.

# Chapter 8: Specialty Soap Making

When you have gotten your feet wet by beginning your cleanser going with the more straightforward formulas you can then proceed onward to claim to fame cleanser making. This kind of soap making can likewise turn out to be savvy when you start to utilize your items on yourself and your family!

For the women, I have a formula for you that is useful for evaluating cosmetics and abandoning your skin feeling spotless and revived. Attempt your hand (and face) at Cool Cream Cleanser and this is all you will require:

4 oz M&P cleanser

Two tsp ice cream

10 drops scent oil

One drop shading (discretionary)

Melt cleanser then includes ice cream and blend

Presently for those of us who appreciate a light botanical aroma, I would exceptionally suggest you make some Citrus and Calendula Cleanser and the supply list incorporates:

One # M and P straightforward cleaner base

A modest bunch of calendula petals (dried), around 1/4 glass

15 drops of yellow sustenance shading

3/4 tsp. grapefruit EO

1/2 tsp. tangerine EO

1 TBSP softened shea butter..melted independently

Initially liquefy the cleanser base and in the meantime soften the shea margarine in a custard container set in a skillet of bubbling water or the microwave. Add calendula petals to the dissolved base, a couple of drops of yellow sustenance shading, the EO and after that the softened shea spread. Attempt to have this the same temp as the melt and pour. Continue mixing the cleanser/shea range blend. As it sets up spoon into heart molds.

(By spooning you have more control what number of the calendula leaves go into every frame.) I get a kick out of the chance to give my images an opportunity to set at room temp until they are skimmed over genuinely firm then I chill them in the cooler for around a half hour before expelling them out the mold and place them on a rack to get done with drying totally. This is an exceptionally alluring cleanser, and this formula will make eight heart soaps.

I can genuinely verify the delight of utilizing Cucumber Loofah Cleanser, and it is not troublesome at all to make. The fixings include:

3 oz. obscure cleanser

Two tsp. Powdered loofah

15 drops cucumber aroma oil

1 T. Aloe Vera gel

green shading

mold

At first, you need to shred the cleanser in a nourishment processor and put aside. Bubble 1/some water over moderate warmth and mix in the destroyed cleanser.

Keep mixing until the blend turns into a sticky mass, roughly four minutes. Expel from heat and mix in the aloe vera gel, the scented oil, and the shading until all around mixed. Spoon the blend into a mold and let set for six hours or until solidified. Wrap completed cleansers in cellophane and appreciate!

There are additionally cleansers that I get a kick out of the chance to make for improvement to be utilized amid the Christmas season and my most loved of all is Nutty cake Cleanser and you will require:

3 - 4oz. Glycerine Cleansers (12 oz)

Sustenance Shading

Scent Oils (Tangerine, Cherry, Pineapple, Lime, Gingerbread and Cinnamon)

You can utilize rectangular cleanser molds, little piece dish or small bundt skillet.

Melt 4 ounces of cleaner and fill 4 square or rectangular soap molds.

Promptly include the accompanying in a specific order:

To start with Mold:

3 drops red sustenance shading and 5 drops Cherry aroma oil

Second Shape:

Two drops red, one drop yellow food shading and 5 drops Tangerine fragrance oil

Third Shape:

Three drops yellow sustenance shading and 5 drops Pineapple aroma oil

Fourth Shape:

Three drops green food shading and 5 drops Lime fragrance oil

Permit the four cleansers to set totally then expel them from the molds and block.

Isolate the solid shaded shapes into cleaner images - recollect that if you are utilizing dish to shower them with a light layer of vegetable splash and wipe out with a paper towel. Melt remaining soap, when softened mix in 1/4 teaspoon Gingerbread aroma oil and 5 drops Cinnamon scent oil.

Include 5 drops caramel sustenance shading or chestnut glue nourishment shading just to make a "nutty surprise" shading. Empty cleanser gradually into molds over the 3D shapes and permit to set for no less than three hours.

Pretty much as the soap is setting mix them to spread the 3D squares around then unmold. On the off chance that you experience difficulty expelling them from the container, utilize a hair dryer to warm the molds marginally.

Once more, It would be simple for you to profit while additionally profiting by hours of pleasure. Be innovative, thought of your Forte cleanser!

# Chapter 9: How To Create Great Recipes

Making a homemade soap recipe is a very creative activity. Your imagination is not limited here, and each piece of soap turns to be a special masterpiece.

Your partner in a magical soap making process is soap calculator or calculator of alkali.

Soap Calc (http://www.soapcalc.net/calc/SoapCalcW P.asp) is convenient because selecting from a list of certain oil, you can see the properties and composition of each oil acids. In addition, you can specify the total weight of the oil immediately (approximately equal to the weight of the ready-made soap), and adjust the amount of each oil from the optional percentage or grams. This calculator also enables to use different fats of animal origin in the recipe. In fact except for vegetable oils, soap can be made of pork, beef, mutton fat, butter, etc.

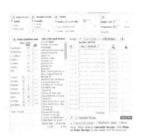

Making the recipe, you need to decide which way you want to make your homemade soap. Soap is brewed in hot or cold way. Everything depends on you and the available time. Cold pulping process takes about an hour, but for the ready soap you should wait at least 3 weeks. Hot pulping process takes you 4-5 hours, but you get the soap ready the next day.

Make sure that soap making cold process is fast enough. Below are the main stages of cooking soap by cold process:

• weigh oils, liquid, alkaline additives;

• melt the oil over a water bath while they were being drown themselves, dilute alkali in the water;

• mix oil and alkali, using a hand blender, until the so-called state of "trace". This state is easy to notice - flowing from the blender, you can write with your finger on the surface of the mass. The soap mass reaches the "trace" state in about 15-20 minutes;

• add essential oils, useful additives, colorants etc.

• fill the molds with the ready mass, wrap them in a cloth or towel and place in a warm place for the night;

• get the soap out of molds the next day, cut if necessary and put to ripe for 3-4 weeks.

Hot pulping process takes about 2-4 hours over a water bath to completely react with the alkali oils. But you can use hot-brewed soap after freezing. Making soap recipe in advance is very important, because it depends on the amount of superfat pointed in the calculator (amount of oils that do not react with alkali, and will have treating properties).

Calculation for making cold process soap

Superfat at cold pulping process is immediately shown on the calculator. Since all oils, irrespective of whether they were added all at once or after a "trace" react in soap making process. Here, for the cold process soap making, superfat is 10%, water - 33%.

The grams are highlighted red.

Selected alkali is highlighted orange.

Water percentage and superfat are highlighted green as well as and the oil weight which are shown manually. Superfat may be different, but for cosmetic soap it is better to use not less than 5-6% (unless you do not make household soap, for which you can take 1-2% superfat. But it is better to lay still "extra amount" superfat, that is, if you want 2% - take 4.3% , etc.).

Show the weight of each oil taken and click "Calculate Recipe".

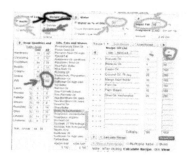

Calculation for making hot process soap

In this case superfat is separately calculated from the total weight of all oils. While calculating it is better to set "extra amount" of superfat of 1-2% (and even 3%). Since the soaping amount of the same oil from different manufacturers may differ, it is better to make calculations on the possible discrepancy of soaping amount, from which this calculation with a soaping value of your oil is derived. Here, for hot pulping method, the superfat is shown by 1% ("extra amount"), the amount of water - 38%. Color codes are the same as for the cold process calculation method.

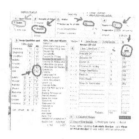

In both cases:

The balanced recipe (INS) **and** the total iodine value **of future soap is highlighted purple.**

**The amount of iodine** shows us the hardness of soap, the lower it is, the harder the soap is. This index should be equal to or less than 55 (it can be a little more, but not too much). Also according to **the amount of iodine** you can determine the expiry date of the soap. The higher it is, the more unsaturated fatty acids exist (mono-and poly-) in the oil (fat), the more it tends to rancidity and oxidation. Such soap produces unpleasant smell and stains like rust.

**Balance.** The balance is better to be about 160 ( 5-6 steps are possible from both sides). If the recipe is well balanced, the soap will be hard enough, with a thick creamy resistant foam and will not dry. This figure does not work for monosoaps (soaps welded with one oil, for example, salt on pure coconut or castile from pure olives), as well as soaps, in which the content of one of the oils is more than 60%.

Other parameters (left column, "Individual Characteristics / Total Data"). **We are interested in the total characteristics of the future soap.**

**Hardness.** The figure is only for solid soap. Good toughness is obtained in the range of 35-50. I should not be confused with an iodine quantity. This indicator is calculated, based on the content of high fatty acids and is responsible for the hardness of soap - myristic, lauric, palmitic and stearic.

**Cleansing.** This figure shows the cleaning properties of the soap. The higher it is, the harder the soap by its function is. Average range - 15-25. If it is below 15, then the cleaning properties will be too weak, in case if it is above 25 it will dry the sensitive skin. For normal skin type, you can exceed this range even if the water is not very hard. This rate is affected by the content of myristic and lauric high fatty acids.

**Conditioning.** An indicator which shows how soft the soap affects on the skin, whether it will dry or not. The normal range is of 50-70. It can be brought up to 80, but foaming will drop then. This Factor is affected by the content of ritsin (which exists only in castor oil), linoleic, linolenic, oleic IVH.

**Foaming.** This value indicates whether the soap will foam well, how lush and large foaming it will produce. The higher the score is, the more blistering it is, and the larger foam bubbles it will make. For good quality foaming the range should be nearly 15-25. It may also be higher, respectively, the foaming properties will be higher. Myristic and lauric acid exert their influence here too, these are responsible not only for cleaning properties, but also for soap foaming. Do not forget about it when choosing the oil.

**Stability / cream foaming.** It shows how stable and creamy the foam will be. Stearic, palmitic and ritsin high fatty acids affect on creaminess and foam stability. The more blistering there is, the less creaminess will be, and vice versa. The usual range for this indicator - 15-35, at higher range, foaming will very creamy, but with little bubbles.

Manual formula calculation

To calculate the required amount of alkali and water, we need to know the quantity of soaping (SAP) of each oil taken. Soaping quantity is initially considered by KOH, it means how many milligrams of hydroxide are needed to soap as many triglycerides high fat acids, and phosphatides, as they exist in 1 gram of a particular fat (vegetable or animal).

To calculate how much sodium hydroxide is needed to soap 1 gram of a particular fat, you must divide potassium number of soaping of the selected oil to 1.40272. The total number can be rounded to three decimal places.

Sample

Potassium number of soaping of palm oil is 0,199. Dividing 0,199 to 1,40272, we can get 0,14186722938291319721683586175431. Round up to 3 after the comma, then we get 0,142.

This number is to soap palm oil for sodium hydroxide.

Now let's calculate how much NaOH we need to soap 200 g of palm oil. 0.142 * 200 = 28.4. Soaping 200 g of palm oil we need 28.4 g of sodium hydroxide.

Similarly, we can count the amount of alkali for each of the selected oil and then summarize. Thus, we obtain the total amount of alkali for the total amount of oils. Superfat wherein is 0%. If we want to calculate superfat for cholesterol, we need to reduce the amount of alkali for the percentage needed.

Take superfat of 10%. Our 28.4 g = 100%. And we need 90% alkali. (28.4 / 100) * 90 = 25.56. That is, our 90% alkali = 25.56 g

Or it can be calculated directly: 0,142 * 200 * 90% = 25.56.

Now we need to calculate the water. If we want to take 33% of water (this is enough for XC, sometimes I take even less), then we need to multiply the mass of oils by 0.33. If it is 38% then it is 0.38, etc. That is, 200 * 0,33 = 66. So we need to take 66 g. of water.

Table of soaping oils and fats

There is the list of coefficients to soap various oils using NaOH (sodium hydroxide) and KOH (potassium hydroxide). From these coefficients one can simply and rapidly determine how much alkali is required for complete soaping of the required amount of oil. To have it completed we simply multiply the oil weight by the coefficient and get the amount of alkali necessary for the complete soaping of the oil quantity.

For example: let's define how much sodium hydroxide is needed for complete soaping of 1 kg of olive oil.

1000 g. of olive oil multiply by the coefficient, according to the table, for

NaOH, i.e for 0.1345 and get: 1000 * 0.1345 = 134.5 g. of NaOH. Calculation of potash soap is made in the same 1000 * 0.18867 = 188.67 g. of KOH. Thus we get the alkali values, which is necessary for soaping a given amount of oil. During soap making it is always advisable to add a little more oil (superfat) for the non-soapened oil to soften the harsh detergent effect of soap. For cold pulping oils of the lowest coefficient of soaping go into the superfat, for hot pulping – take any you wish: you should add these after the soap turns into gel.

The amount of iodine indicates the content of double bonds in oils and fats, it determines the overall non saturation of oils and fats. The higher the iodine value the more non saturated fatty acids are contained in the fat, i.e. more iodine substance can be added.

In terms of the soap iodine amount one can roughly estimate the hardness of soap (for solid soaps indicator must be over 55) as well as how long it will be kept. The harder the soap, the longer it is kept and is not rancid, i.e. does not oxidize during storage.

| Oil | Coefficient for NaOH | Coefficient for KOH | Iodine value |
|---|---|---|---|
| Avocado | 0,1335 | 0,18726 | 12-20 |
| Annatto | 0,1330 | 0,18656 | 103-115 |
| Peanut | 0,1355 | 0,19007 | 148-157 |
| Apricot kernel | 0,1350 | 0,18937 | 92-108 |
| Argan | 0,1360 | 0,19077 | 80-95 |
| Babassu | 0,1750 | 0,24548 | 10-12 |

| | | | |
|---|---|---|---|
| Grape seed | 0,1285 | 0,18025 | 125-142 |
| Walnut | 0,1335 | 0,18726 | 140-150 |
| Shea | 0,1282 | 0,17983 | 55-71 |
| Jojoba | 0,0660 | 0,09258 | 33-42 |
| Wheat germ | 0,1310 | 0,18376 | 125-135 |
| Rice germ | 0,1345 | 0,18867 | 98-110 |
| Corn | 0,1360 | 0,19077 | 93-106 |
| Pumpkin seed | 0,1350 | 0,18937 | 28-36 |
| Cocoa | 0,1380 | 0,19358 | 6-11 |
| Camellia | 0,1360 | 0,19077 | 6-10 |
| Castor | 0,1286 | 0,18039 | 82-90 |
| Coconut | 0,1830 | 0,2567 | 114- |

| | | | |
|---|---|---|---|
| | | | 150 |
| Hemp | 0,1345 | 0,18867 | 90-103 |
| Sesame | 0,1376 | 0,19301 | 105-115 |
| Laurel | 0,1405 | 0,19708 | 170-180 |
| Lanolin | 0,0750 | 0,1052 | 18-36 |
| Linseed oil | 0,1340 | 0,18796 | 74-78 |
| Hazelnut oil | 0,1370 | 0,19217 | 80-85 |
| Poppy | 0,1383 | 0,194 | 132-136 |
| Macadamia | 0,1390 | 0,19498 | 103-130 |
| Mango | 0,1339 | 0,18782 | 124 |
| Passionfruit | 0,1290 | 0,18095 | 125-140 |

| | | | |
|---|---|---|---|
| Black cumin oil | 0,1350 | 0,18937 | 122-126 |
| Almond | 0,1365 | 0,19147 | 54-66 |
| Olive | 0,1345 | 0,18867 | 77-90 |
| Oenothera biennis | 0,1345 | 0,18867 | 145-162 |
| Palm oil | 0,1405 | 0,19708 | 50-58 |
| Peach kernel | 0,1345 | 0,18867 | 108-118 |
| Sunflower | 0,1350 | 0,18937 | 122-138 |
| Safflower | 0,1355 | 0,19007 | 85-105 |
| Soybean | 0,1355 | 0,19007 | 124-132 |
| Rosehip | 0,1359 | 0,19063 | 180-195 |
| Duck fat | 0,138 | 0,193 | 72 |

| | | | |
|---|---|---|---|
| Pork fat | 0,141 | 0,198 | 57 |
| Sheep fat | 0,138 | 0,193 | 54 |
| Goose fat | 0,137 | 0,192 | 65 |
| Beef tallow | 0,143 | 0,200 | 45 |
| Butterfat | 0,255 | 0,357 | 16-19 |
| Chicken fat | 0,139 | 0,195 | 69 |
| Bees wax | 0,0690 | 0,09679 | 86-91 |
| Carnauba wax | 0,0690 | 0,09679 | 86-119 |
| Palm stearin | 0,1460 | 0,2048 | 2-3 |

Useful soap additives

Besides treating, conditioning oils there are many other components that can be added during homemade soap making. They not only enrich your handmade soaps with new properties, but also change the daily shower or bath habits.

Let's call these components as useful additive.

These include:

• **milk**: cow, goat, mare, almond, coconut, etc. Milk enriches soap with delicate texture.

Milk can replace some or all of the water in which you dilute alkali. For these purposes, you must first freeze it to avoid unpleasant odor and color changes in the interacting with alkali.

Dry milk is also added into the superfat. Use up to 10% of all superfatting ingredients. The fat content of milk powder should be taken into consideration and subtract its amount from the total weight of oils for superfat. For example, you decided that you need 50 g of oil for superfat. You want to add 10% of dry milk of 25% fat into superfat. Thus 10% - is 5 g., and considering that the milk fat is 25%, it is necessary to take four times more, i.e. 20g.

Thus 20 g. of milk powder will contain 5 g. of fat, which becomes part of superfat. Accordingly you will have to add 45 g. of the rest superfatting components.

• **yogurt**: Use natural plain yogurt without additives and sugar. At cold soap pulping process dissolve yogurt in the liquid for cooking alkaline solution and freeze, at the hot pulping process add yogurt partially during cooking or at the last stage.

• **honey**: has moisturizing properties, helps to increase the volume of foam soap. At cold soap pulping process, add the melted honey into the ready cooled alkaline solution or mix with major oils, at hot pulping process- before putting it into the mold. For 500 g of oil 1 tablespoon of honey is needed.

• **sugar**: promotes soap foaming, colors the soap brown. Use up to 1 tsp. for 500 g of oil.

• **fructose**: increases the stability of the foam in the soap. For 500 g of oil, add 1 tablespoon of fructose.

• **beeswax**: provides soap with hardness. Blend wax with major oils, for this first melt the wax (wax melting point is 60-65 ° C), then add the rest of the solid oil to it and continue to heat up. Use up to 5% in the soap.

• **cereal** (whole or ground): nourishes the skin, gives the effect of peeling and interesting texture. It is perfect for milk-honey soap.

• **flour, corn starch**: gives tender texture to the soap.

• **fruits and vegetables, berries and herbs**: lemon, orange, grapefruit, tangerine, banana, strawberry, apple, pear, cucumber, carrots, beets, onions, parsley ... use everything you can find in the kitchen.

It is much more interesting to use juice, as alkali can burn the pulp, besides soap with fresh vegetable or fruit puree becomes fast rotten and its expiry date is short. Do not add more than 10% of puree. Juice from fruits, vegetables, greens and herbs can be used to prepare the alkaline solution, and also add at the trace stage.

Use dried fruit slices for soap decoration. Citrus is especially popular for this purpose. Cut the fruit into thin slices and let them aside for a couple of months in the sun or dry them in the oven for about 8 hours.

• **acids in the soap**: requires an additional amount of alkali. The acid is first diluted in a small amount of liquid, and then carefully added to the ready alkaline solution.

**Citric acid** reacting with alkali in the soap forms sodium citrate, which softens hard water. Soap with citric acid has the additional conditioning effect. For this reason, the citric acid is one of the indispensable additives into the shampoo soap. Citric acid input percentage in the soap: 0.1-1.0% of the total weight of the oils. For 1 g of citric acid, some 0.6 g of additional alkali is necessary.

**Lactic acid** forms sodium lactate in the soap, which has an antibacterial effect, is a powerful moisturizer, restores damaged lipid layer of the skin and treats dehydrated skin. Soap, made with the additional sodium lactate does not dry even sensitive, prone to allergies, skin. The lactic acid soap is more solid and smooth, i.e. acquires the so called "trademark" look. To neutralize 1 g of 80% lactic acid it is necessary to add an additional 0.36 g of alkali. Input of lactic acid into soap: up to 3%. The combination of lactic acid and

92

fruit, berry juice peels and flattens the skin tone, and has a lifting effect.

**Stearic acid** gives the soap hardness, increases the stability of foam, gives dullness,speeds up the "trace". When interacting with alkali it forms sodium stearate, which enhances the activity of acting ingredients in soap. 3-5% is used in soap and increases the stability of the foam.

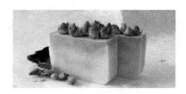

• **flowers and petals** (dried or fresh): calendula, chamomile, lavender, rose, heather. Use also plant extracts and infusions (oil infused with herbs).

Dried flowers, petals, herbs can be used for soap décor: sprinkle them on the soap just after placing in the mold. Chopped herbs are suitable for scrub or peeling effect. For giving their useful properties much better, dried flowers and herbs, fill them with warm oil for superfat beforehand and then add to the soap with these oils.

For dyeing soap into the yellow color, use petals of marigold or dandelion grounded in a blender or cut with knife.

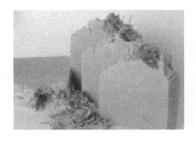

• **silk**: nourishes the skin, making it smooth and elastic. Input percentage 5-10%. Silk is added to the alkaline solution. Liquid silk begins to thicken, so add it gradually.

• **menthol**: input percentage 1.5-5%. Menthol Soap is very refreshing in the morning or on hot day. Menthol dissolves in oils, so it's better to melt it with butter.

• **clay**: gives useful properties to the skin. Clay absorbs toxins, normalizes metabolic processes in the skin, improves blood circulation. Use colored clay as a natural colorant for soap. Clays are pink, green, yellow, red, blue. Paints obtained here are slightly muted and the soap looks very natural. Clay should be diluted beforehand in a little water or oil, to avoid lumps.

• **sea salt**: tightens skin, increases blood flow, makes soap harder; added in large quantities it dries the skin. Use up to 2 tsp. sea salt per 500 g of oils.

• **essential oils and flavorings**: significantly speeds up the start of the "trace", consider this fact when you make soap with swirls. input percentage: from 1% to 4% from weight of oils.

Of course, if you've already decided to make soap from scratch, to make it 100% natural it is better not to use artificial fragrances and use natural essential oils to give flavor to soap. Besides the wonderful aroma of essential oils they will give your soap useful properties from the heart of the plant. Not to hurt your skin and avoid allergy, use only 100% natural essential oils. The use of artificial and synthetic essential oils is appropriate and justified only in perfumery to create original perfumes, but unacceptable for creating useful and natural product - that is, your homemade soap.

If you are prone to allergies, it is better to totally refuse using essential oils and flavors in any soap.

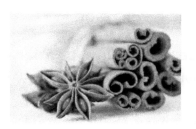

• **spices**: provide soap with useful and healing properties, many of the spices are a great natural dye for the soap from scratch. Add spices in fresh or dried ground form, together with superfat and use for décor (asterisk star anise, clove buds, cinnamon sticks, bay leaf, peppercorns, etc.).

**Ginger**: tones, moisturizes. Use ground ginger, fresh grated ginger or fresh ginger juice.

**Parsley**: dyes soap in green. Use juice or fresh chopped herbs in a blender.

**Rosemary**: improves blood circulation to the skin. Preserves its fragrance in soaps.

**Sage**: Fresh herbs provide soap with fragrance and green color.

**Saffron**: use as a yellow powder or dried flowers. Gives soap natural yellow color.

**Curry**: makes soap yellow.

**Paprika**: gives soap reddish hues.

**Turmeric**: is responsible for peach tones.

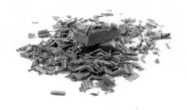

• **cocoa mass**: gives soap chocolate color and flavor, provides moisturizing and caring effect, due to the content of cocoa oil in it. Use in soap up to 5%, for the foam not stain brown. Add as superfat, but take into consideration the fact that fat of cocoa mass is 50%, hence, you should reduce the amount of other superfat components to 25%. For example, the total oil weight is 1000g , make soap with superfat of 10%. For superfat, in addition, take 5% of cocoa mass - 50 g Subtract 25% out of oil weights for superfat (100 g)  - the remaining 75 g are superfat components (oils).

• **cocoa powder**: is used for coloring soap in shades of brown.

• **birch tar**: it turns homemade soap into the real medicine. The tar is widely used in folk medicine due to its strong antiseptic, antipruritic and anti-inflammatory properties. Tar soap will help you quickly and effectively to deal with skin and hair problems such as dandruff, itching, psoriasis, eczema, ringworm, dries pimples, makes hair soft and silky. Input percentage of tar in soap is 1-10%.

# Chapter 10: Stay Clean Respecting Nature

Cleaning your home and office is important in respect for the people who live inside it; but how important is it to do it also respecting the environment? Recently the attention to ecology, the environment in which we live, the ecosystem, is subject of great social and civil impact, so much so that even the world of cleaning companies is changing and also the cleaning products we use.

Unfortunately, it is well-known that household and professional cleaning products are often polluting and harmful to the surrounding environment, so much so that ecologists have always raised strong controversies and campaigns precisely against the use of these detergents.

Our house, especially if inhabited by children, is often dirty and untidy. The need for cleaning is mandatory, above all to prevent children from being contaminated by bacteria and other types of microorganisms that are enemies of health.

To try to clean deeply, we often can make mistakes of using very aggressive detergent products, with the presence of surfactants, which facilitate cleaning and remove stubborn dirt.

Unfortunately, these detergents are highly polluting and despite rinsing, they remain attached to the floor and therefore in contact with our skin. In the hope of cleaning well, we risk doing even more damage to health, as well as to the external environment.

Ecological products, on the other hand, are formulated with ingredients of plant origin and exploit essential oils and antiseptic properties from nature.

The presence of soluble oils, vegetable substances and salts dissolved in water, allows to obtain a deep cleaning, in maximum safety for health.

Many people, because of their commitments, are unable to dedicate time to the eco-sustainable cleaning of their home and therefore, going to the supermarket, they buy what they find, perhaps the cheapest product probably with a very high environmental impact. According to recent statistics, the production of chemicals in Europe is 33% and between 15 and 20 chemicals that an average family uses at home for a total of about 400 million tons of chemicals produced from 1930 until today.

The renewed interest in the respect and care of the environment around us, has meant that many companies of products to be used for cleaning, have started to create and market products that are completely green, non-polluting and made with completely natural ingredients. Choosing an eco-friendly product does not mean that the latter has a poor cleaning and sanitizing action, indeed, these type of green products have nothing to envy to strong and polluting products.

On the rise in supermarkets, we find many bottles or draft detergents, highly recommended for the respect of the environment: buying the empty bottle only once, we can always use it, paying only the refill of detergent, thus saving about 50 - 60 %, avoiding plastic waste.

But if you want to completely eliminate the impact caused by household cleaning products, and at the same time keep the rooms sanitized, the alternatives exist and your grandmothers will be able to confirm it to you! We would like to keep an eye also on another way to keep in good health and practice good hygiene:

3.1 Essential oils

Essential oils can be defined as natural compounds of plant origin made up of mixtures of volatile substances at room temperature. In other words, essential oil is not constituted by a single molecule, but by a mixture of different molecules, generally of a terpenic nature. Essential oils or essences are natural compounds of plant oils that are characterized by the presence of volatile substances that give the product different smells and fragrances. It is no coincidence, therefore, that essential oils are also known as "volatile oils".

Characteristics and properties of each essential oil may vary according to the mixture that constitutes it. However, it is possible to identify some characteristics common to all essential oils. From a chemical point of view, these substances are characterized by marked volatility (presence of low boiling compounds) and a composition based mostly on compounds having low molecular weight.

From a biological point of view, however, essential oils are characterized by being produced from specific cells and then poured out, or collected in specialized spaces and specific organoleptic characteristics.

## 3.2 Nasal Irrigation

It can effectively and quickly restore the functionality of the mucous membrane of the nose, restoring its purifying, humidifying and immune function. The activity of nasal washing does not just clean and free the nasal pits from the accumulation of secretions, but also performs a decongestant action, increasing the passage of air inside the nasal cavities and alleviating the typical unpleasant sensation of the nose "closed".

In this way, the well-being of the individual is obtained by perfecting nasal breathing and, consequently, promoting the best functionality of the lower respiratory tract.

This technique has ancient origins. For thousands of years, in the Yoga tradition, nasal pits have been cleaned with saline solutions. As you know, the goal of Yoga philosophy is to connect the body and soul with God to obtain the state of psycho-physical well-being. For this purpose, meticulous attention is paid to breathing techniques. It is in this context that the practice of JalaNeti takes place, that is, to run a saline solution into the nose using an ampoule called Lota resting on the nostril that you want to cleanse.

3.3 Propolis Spray

The propolis used is naturally produced by bees, without forced production techniques. Used as an antiseptic and defense substance for the hive, it has a very unique and agreeable smell, very similar to that of honey with the addition of strong balsamic notes.

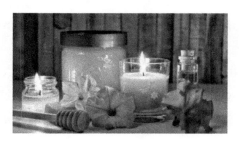

Propolis is made up of numerous natural, assorted substances, the percentage of which is highly unpredictable depending on the seasons and the type of plants around the hive. It contains a high content of flavonoids (in particular galantine), tannins, coffee acid and essential oils which donate to the physiological well-being of the throat.

### 3.4 Vitamins

The food normally included in the diet, in general, do not correspond to good sources of vitamin D. However, regular utilization of those that are richer in them can, in part, help offset the insufficient production of vitamin D3 by the skin in periods of less exposure to the sun, such as in winter or when you cannot spend enough time in the open air during the day due to diseases, unfavorable weather conditions, professional commitments, etc.

Among the foods that contain the greatest quantities of vitamin D we mention: some types of fish like salmon, herring, mackerel, sardines and in general all the fish of the North Seas- also rich in omega-3 fats beneficial for the nervous system and cardiovascular system, pig's liver, whole milk and yogurt, butter, fatty cheeses, eggs, milk and / or egg-based creams. Marseille soap is a 100% natural product based on vegetable oils and sometimes essential oils useful for the care of the body, face and hair thanks to the remarkable properties it has.

## 3.5 Wash your clothes with natural ingredients

Often washing clothes in the washing machine is not adequate to have your clothes completely safe and sanitized. Often the use of chemicals can cause allergies and dermatitis and, as they are not biodegradable, they also cause pollution. We want to show you some easy remedies for disinfecting and sanitizing your laundry.

### 3.5.1 Lemon

Lemon is an excellent friend for disinfecting and perfuming laundry. Just add a few drops to the detergent by hand or in the washing machine.

If you have soft and delicate woolen items, simply leave them to soak for a day in a solution of water and lemon juice (2 lemons per liter of water). In order not to make the garments yellow, simply immerse the clothes in a tray with cold water and the juice of two lemons and leave them to soak for about an hour. To revive the silk, however, just wash it with soap, rinse it and leave it to soak for a few hours in water and lemon juice.

### 3.5.2 Sodium per-carbonate

Sodium per-carbonate is an excellent whitening, totally natural that also has powerful sanitizing properties. It comes in granular form and acts thanks to the presence of oxygen and can eliminate even the most stubborn stains. If you are going to do a whitening wash thoroughly, add a spoonful of per-carbonate and wash at 60 ° C, the temperature at which this compound becomes more effective. You can do the 60-degree test with or without per-carbonate and the difference is noticeable.

In the case of a normal wash, you can do exactly the same, but you only need tousle a spoonful of sodium per-carbonate and set the temperature of the washing machine to 40ºC.

But be aware that it is not suitable for delicate clothes like wool, silk or leather. It does not pollute, and it does not contain enzymes, surfactants, optical brighteners, nor phosphorus nor allergens.

### 3.5.3 Vinegar

Vinegar is a good disinfectant, as well as degreasing and deodorant. Suitable for removing stains, even the most stubborn ones, and fixing colors at the first wash. Just put the clothes to soak in a bowl containing hot water and half a cup of white vinegar. After one night it will be sufficient to wash them as usual.

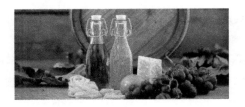

The vinegar used during the rinse phase is also an excellent anti-lime scale that makes the washing machine last longer or, used in place of the softener, prevents detergent and limestone "hardening" the fibers of the fabrics leaving them soft to the touch.

Adding half a cup of vinegar directly when doing a wash increases the cleaning power of the detergent itself, making the colors more intense and bright. It also removes the halos of deodorants from clothing and eliminates bad smells, especially those of the kitchen and cigarette. Furthermore, if you add the vinegar to the normal washing cycle, it will be able to rid the garments of animal hair.

### 3.5.4 Tea tree oil

Tea Tree essential oil has known antibacterial, healing, antifungal, and anti-odor properties. It is an extract of the leaves of the Melaleuca tree and is an excellent solution for sanitizing and perfuming laundry, being a powerful natural disinfectant.

Just add 4-5 drops to the detergent. To have a do-it-yourself disinfectant, you can put a tablespoon of tea tree oil in a liter bottle of white alcohol for liquor, leave it to rest for a week in a dark bottle and then use it in the wash, adding 1 or 2 tablespoons for every 5 kilos of laundry

# Chapter 11: Soap Making Methods

There are many methods to make soap, some are quite easy while others are an art; a complex art, but not impossible.

Melt and pour method

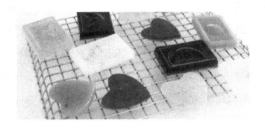

This is one of the easiest soap making processes and saves quite a lot of time. In this process, you can use a premade soap base that has undergone the saponification process rather than spend time mixing fats with an alkali such as lye, which can be time consuming as it requires more preparation time. A readymade soap base contains glycerin and fatty acids as well as other natural ingredients.

The melt and pour method is the perfect choice if you are a beginner, still exploring the arena and would like to play it safe. All you have to do is purchase pre-made solid soap base instead of making it from scratch and you are ready to use the soap once it hardens, no unnecessary waiting for a cure time to pass such as with cold process.

How this method works:

Head to a nearby arts and crafts store and look for a premade soap base. One of the best options to purchase are the clear glycerin or white premade soap bases. Don't use a bar of soap for this as it is not the same thing and will give you trouble while melting.

The next step would be to melt your solid premade soap base. To speed up this process, use a sharpened knife to cut the bar into small 1-inch chunks. Don't worry about exact measurements here. The goal is to have smaller pieces rather than one large chunk as smaller pieces will melt faster.

In a microwave, add your cut chunks in a microwave friendly dish and heat for 30 seconds. Take out the dish and stir your melted contents then reheat again for another 30 seconds then take out to stir again. Repeat this cycle of 30 seconds heat then stir until you feel the consistency of your melted soap base as completely liquidy with no lumps or hard chunks in between. That is when your entire soap base has melted. Don't overheat it beyond that point.

Some people don't own a microwave in their house, it is possible to replace it with a saucepan filled with water to create a water bath. Heat the water and then put a glass bowl and let it float in the hot water.

Put your soap base chunks in the glass bowl and watch it melt through the heat that transfers from the hot water to the glass bowl and consequently to the soap base chunks that melt eloquently. Don't forget to stir. Remove the bowl from the sauce pan when your soap base has completely melted and doesn't have any lumps.

Let your soap melt to cool down to around 50 degree Celsius. Do not add your essential oils or dye while the melt is still hot. Likewise, don't let it cool to the point of hardening. Add 2-3 drops of your desired dye depending on the color intensity you desire. If you are using a powdered dye, dissolve 2-3 teaspoons of your powdered dye in some liquid glycerin as you can't add the power directly to your melt or else the color will not get distributed evenly. It is always wonderful to add a pleasant scent to your soap. For 1 pound of soap, you can add 1 tablespoon of fragrance oil or half a tablespoon of

117

essential oil. Make sure you use the ones labelled for soap making and not candle oils, to ensure they are friendly and soft on your skin.

Stir all your added dye and fragrance drops before the last step. The last step would be to pour your colored and fragranced melt into a mold of your choice then let it cool naturally for 12-24 hours. When your soap has completely solidified, take it out of the mold and it would be ready for use immediately. However, make sure the edges have dried completely.

The rebatching method

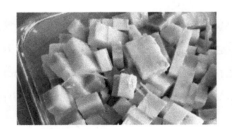

A similar quick and easy method is the rebatching method. As the name suggests, it is often used to rebatch (make use of the soap you did) if there were any mistakes or if you didn't like the shape of the mold or messed it up during the design process. You can also use this method if you want to get a taste of the soap making DIY experience without buying additional equipment. In that cause, you can use pre existing soap. However, readymade soap never melts easily, that is why, although you will heat it as we described in the melt and pour method, you will add few table spoons of water, glycerin, etc to soften up the mix, then with heat resistant gloves, you will add your soap melt in a Ziploc bag and knead it so make it into a mushy texture.

Similar to the melt and pour process, you can add the dye and fragrance to your mix in the rebatching method and then let it solidify. This will take 5-7 days however as you wait for all the water to evaporate.

Don't get impatient and use the freezer. Rebatched soap does not have the most aesthetic look or feel, but it is a suitable solution to ruined soap or if you want to add your own color and fragrance to existing soap. Moreover, this method bypasses the drawback of adding stuff that get ruined by lye such as lavender buds that turn brown with lye. You can also use colors that are sensitive to the pH of lye that you can't use in the cold process. Similar is the case with being able to use light fragrances with the rebatching method which get masked when used in the cold process.

The benefits of both rebatching and melt and pour methods is that you don't have to deal with lye, which is feared by many people as it is a strong alkali. Moreover, you don't even need a lot of ingredients to start with or complex calculations and you can immediately get to enjoying the soap once it solidifies. However, on the other hand, you have very little control over the raw ingredients used as you are starting with something that someone else made, you don't control everything from scratch as with the cold method. If you would like to be the master of the experiment and totally in control of what goes in your soap, then the cold process is the best process for you.

The hot process

This process is like the cold process but involves using heat pots and "cooking" the soap rather than doing it cold.

The cold process

Keep in mind that in soap making, the cold process is the dragon level of all levels. The game play becomes a little bit more complex, but don't worry we have got your back and we are here to guide you through it step by step. The reward here is that there are unlimited possibilities to how you can make your final product in terms of colors, shapes and natural additions. Moreover, you can 100% guarantee that your soap is home made from scratch.

Let us start with the basic ingredients you will need for making soap using the cold process:

Lye flakes and clean distilled water

A source of fat, whether animal fat or vegetable oil

A natural soap dye of your choice, whether liquid or powder (optional but preferred)

Soap pot along with other equipments which we will discuss in more details shortly

Fragrance or an essential oil of your choice (optional but preferred)

A mold of your desired shape

A clean environment to work in and a cool dry place to let the soap cure in

For aesthetics petals or exfoliates (optional)

A handy recipe to follow (we will provide you with one)

How it works:

The essence of the cold soap making process is preparing lye and a source of fat and mixing it together

Making the lye solution

The first step is to prepare the lye solution. For exact amounts, you will have to refer to your chosen recipe.

Using your kitchen scale or digital scale, place the glass pitcher and set the scale to zero. Next you would be adding distilled water as per indicated in your recipe. Some recipes indicate weight; therefore you will place the pitcher on the scale.

Other recipes indicate volume; therefore you can use your measuring cup.

Next it is time to measure up the lye. Do so using your mason jar with a tight secure lid. Lye is an alkali and is dangerous to your skin. That is why you need to handle it using gloves and while wearing your safety goggles. If any lye flakes cling to your glove, remove them immediately. Place the Mason jar and its lid on the scale and set it to zero. Add in the lye flakes until the scale indicates the weight indicated in your chosen recipe. You can replace the Mason jar with a plastic pitcher. However, don't use this pitcher for anything else except handling lye during your soap making process.

After your weights are set as per indicated in your recipe, time to mix them up. But be careful about this step. Take care to add the lye to the water bit by bit and not pour the water to the lye. Gently start adding your lye flakes to the pitcher containing water. Add it bit by bit from a close but safe distance to avoid splashes. To dissolve the lye appropriately, stir the mixture gently and slowly, again without splashing. As the two react, you will start to hear fizzing sounds or feel heat which is normal. Don't let the solution touch your skin directly. Keep your goggles and gloves on. Wash the item you used to stir with immediately after stirring. Don't forget to cover your pitcher containing your newly mixed lye water and let it settle for some time. Make sure it is tied securely and placed in a safe place away from pets or children. Caution should always be in mind around lye or lye water.

Preparing the oils

Get your handy scale again because we will weigh out your chosen oil as per the recipe, using the same method of adding the soap pot or a glass pitcher on the scale and setting it to zero. It is preferred to use the soap pot to weigh solid oils such as cocoa butter while using the glass pitcher for liquid oil such as olive oil. Slowly add the oil to your container till the scale hits the desired weight.

Examples of solid fat sources: Cocoa butter, coconut or palm

Examples of liquid fat sources: Castor oil, canola oil, olive oil, sunflower oil

If you are using a solid oil, melt it first using a sauce pan. This will shorten the step for you as you need to heat your chosen oil anyway. The oil needs to heat gradually, so apply medium heat and stir gently. You need to watch the temperature of your oil using the thermometer and turn off the heat when it reaches about 110 F. However, you can't add it just yet to the lye water mixture. The oils temperature needs to drop to 100 F before it can be mixed with the lye water. If you are using solid oil, make sure all the solid oil has come to a melt. If your recipe indicates a mixture of solid and liquid oils, add the liquid oils after all the solid fats melts. However, monitor your temperature again as this will lower the temperature of the overall oil mixture. Remember, you need it to be around 100 F when you mix it with the lye water.

Add the lye water to the oil base

Once you mix these two, the saponification reaction will be instant, and the mixture will turn cloudy, indicating a chemical reaction where the lye and oil react in the presence of heat to make soap. The lye is no longer chemically lye that is why handmade soap is safe on the skin, it no longer contains lye as it all transformed to soap when it mixed with the hot oil. Because from here on the process will happen quickly, you need to have your desired additions on standby, for example your fragrance bottles, essential oils, dye, spatulas, etc.

Gently add the lye mixture to the hot oil in the soap pot. You will notice a color change and that the mixture will start to be cloudy. Stir gently, preferably with a stick blender, although, keep it turned off at this point. After you have poured in all your lye water mixture, keep the glass pitcher that contained it in a safe spot for the time being until you safely clean it later. Right now, you need to stay with your new mixture.

If you are using a stick blender, turn it on now and let it mix the mixture in short bursts of a few seconds and repeat until you feel that both your lye water and oil have completely mixed until you reach trace. Trace is reached when the mixture has emulsified, meaning, when the mixture is left later, it will keep getting thicker and thicker with time as part of the process.

How to know if you have reached trace point?

The stick blender has severely quickened the process of saponification and reaching trace takes seconds compared to hours using regular stirring. If your mixture still has glistening oily liquidly floating between strokes, then all the oil has not mixed completely with your lye water yet. You will reach trace when the creamy consistency starts to slightly thicken and has a uniform consistency instead of having both thick and oily consistencies.

Why is it important to reach trace point?

For many reasons, chief among them is that since tracing point is the point where all the mixture has emulsified and became soap particles instead of oil and lye, that means pouring the mixture before achieving trace results in having incomplete soap. This will lead to deformed soap or incompletely formed soap. Moreover, you will still have lye particles in your soap which will be very harmful to your skin. Therefore, you need to keep stirring until you have a think cake-like batter consistency with no glistening oil streaks. This mixture will also be easy to pour into a mold and will be of uniform consistency, you won't find oil dripping from the batter

It is safe to add your dye and fragrance in the light trace step before the thick medium trace step begins. Medium trace has a thicker consistency than light trace, resembling that of a pudding consistency. You can test for it by trickling some of the batter from the blender and it will form visible soap streaks on the mixture's surface the way chocolate streaks on a cake. This is the most suitable time to add your natural hard additives such as leaves, exfoliate, petals, etc.

The final trace consistency is that which resembles a thick pudding batter. That is the trace consistency that will conform to its shape when poured into a mold and that is what you want. To reach this trace stage, you need to keep stirring with the stick blender. If you want to create soap frosting, you will need to extremely thicken your trace to get soap consistency for frosting or decorative purposes.

Keep in mind a very important false trace sign. When you use a solid trace, if it has not been thoroughly melted and heating, it can easily cool during the mixing process and give the false sensation of hardening mixture while in fact it is not hardening due to saponification but it is due to hardening of the solid fat. For that reason, make sure to adequately heat it.

Factors that can affect trace consistency

There is no doubt that using a stick will make you reach a medium and thick consistency trace faster than stirring by hand. If you would like to give your dye and fragrance some time to mix, consider stirring by hand using a spatula when you reach thin trace consistency.

Some fragrances and additives such as clay speed up the trace process and make your mixture thicken fast. Be mindful about such additions and the timing and method of stirring. It is preferred to switch to manual stirring after adding a fragrance.

Adding your personal touch to the batter

After reaching your desired state, and before it is too thick, you can now add your chosen fragrance, essential oils and additives such as herbs, petals or natural exfoliants. Then gently stir and make sure your additions are thoroughly mixed within the batter. We will discuss some examples of exfoliants and essential oils.

Coloring your soap

One of the most beautiful aspects of making your own soap is that you can choose the color of your soap. You can have your color as one solid color for the entire bar or you can get creative with color streaks. If you want to have a simply colored bar of soap, add your desired color dye, few drops or ½ a tea spoon into the batter. Make sure it is soap dye and not candle dye. You can add more dye to increase the color intensity of the soap but don't overdo it. Stir well to evenly distribute the color.

If you want to try creative methods such as the streak method, get about half a cup or a cup of your soap separately in your measuring cup and add the dye to it and mix thoroughly. Put the rest of your soap batter in your desired mold and gently pour your colored mixture to the corner of the mold. Using a wooden or rubber spatula, start pulling colored streaks from the colored corner to design the soap batter that is lying in the mold away from the corner. You can swirl around the color to create your desired pattered but don't overdo it so that you don't blend the color with the entire mixture. You can use a Lazy Susan to try swirling techniques. The beauty of this step is that you can get very creative with color designs and patterns or even color combinations of your choice.

Pour your mixture into a mold

By now, your mixture is ready to be poured into your desired mold. As you would evenly pour a cake mix into a mold, do so with your soap batter. A handy rubber spatula will aid you to scrape off the rest of the soap batter in your soap pot and into the mold. Finally, shake the mold gently to evenly distribute the soap batter in your mold to get a uniform bar. To get a soap bar with a smooth surface, you need to smooth out the surface of the mixture and even it out with the back of a spoon or with a rubber spatula.

Sometimes air bubbles would accumulate in your mixture during the pouring step. You will need to get rid of those. Gently tap your mold against the kitchen top to release any bubbles. Finally, leave your soap to cure in a warm and a safe place.

Now it is time to leave your mold for about 24 hours to harden. After this period of time, it would be ready to take it out of the mold and slice it into acceptable size bars. It is best to keep those bars to cure for 4 weeks before using it although it is safe to use right away. Meanwhile, don't forget to wash all the equipment you used very well with hot water and soap while still wearing your gloves and goggles.

# Chapter 12: Basic Equipment And Ingredients Needed

INGREDIENTS

Antioxidant

Antioxidants are an optional ingredient that will extend the life of your soap. I'd recommend rosemary oleoresin extract.

Crock Pot

A crock pot is handy when making hot process soap. A double boiler method also works well for this method, so use whatever is convenient.

Oils

Different oils have different effects on your soap. Olive oil and shea butter are moisturizing, coconut oil has good lather, and palm oil creates a firm bar. There are a few other oils, but these are the most basic that you'll be using in your first soaps. Most homemade soaps will contain a combination of oils, so it's best to follow a recipe first before experimenting with your own different proportions of oils.

Lye

Also known as sodium hydroxide, lye is what makes soap, soap! You can purchase lye from some supermarkets and hardware stores, but it has become increasingly difficult to find. Most lye is not labeled for soap making and is instead used as a drain cleaner. Make sure that if you do find lye from these sources that it is 100% sodium hydroxide! Buying lye online for soap making is also a great option.

Scent

You can choose to leave your soap unscented, or you can add small quantities of essential oils or fragrance oils to scent your home made soap.

## Water

Water plays an important role in the chemical processing of lye. Make sure that you don't use hard water for cold process soap making, as some of the minerals could react with the lye. I recommend using distilled water.

## EQUIPMENT

### Immersion blender

An immersion blender, also known as a stick blender, will ensure a smooth and consistent result. An immersion blender is not required, but will turn strenuous stirring into a few minutes' work.

### Scale

It is important to measure all of your ingredients by weight, especially for small batches of soap. Digital scales are easy to read and can be used for precise baking.

### Stainless Steel Pot

Lye will react with a cast iron, nonstick, or aluminum pot, so make sure to use a stainless steel or enamel-covered pot for making your soap.

Bowls/Containers

It's always helpful to have a variety of bowls and containers for both measuring and mixing. At least one of these bowls should be heat resistant for working with hot materials, so look for a bowl that is stainless steel or pyrex. Don't forget that lye will react with aluminum! Do not use wood bowls, either. Wood can absorb dangerous chemicals.

Drying Rack

Drying racks are important to assist with airflow when soap is curing.

pH Testing Kit

You may want to test the pH of your earliest soaps to make sure they are not too basic.

## Spoons

You'll want to have measuring spoons and mixing spoons on hand. Do not use a wooden spoon.

## Thermometer

It's important to keep track of what temperature your soap mixture is to create the right balance in your soap. More than one thermometer will simplify your process. More on the two thermometers later!

## Soap Mold

A soap mold can be any container. You can use a wood or plastic box, or even a milk carton! Soap molds in pretty shapes are also an option and can be purchased or made at home. I'll show you how to make some further on in the book.

## Freezer Paper

Line your soap molds with freezer paper to prevent sticking.

## Cardboard Box

If you can, find a box that is large enough to cover your soap mold.

## Knife

Any old kitchen knife with a large blade will do the trick.

## Glasses and Gloves

These two pieces of equipment are essential when dealing with lye. Handling lye is completely safe when done correctly, so be sure to wear rubber gloves to protect your hands and goggles or safety glasses to protect your eyes.

## General Safety Guidelines

The importance of safety cannot be stressed enough when making soap. Though making soap at home can be easy and fun, working with chemicals and mixing ingredients over heat warrants some caution. Don't forget your gloves and goggles when you're dealing with lye, and be careful when handling hot ingredients and tools! It is also recommended to wear closed-toe shoes, and avoid a lot of exposed skin on your arms and legs. If you're making soap indoors, be sure to open a few windows to keep the room ventilated. You should also keep a bottle of vinegar handy in case you spill any lye, as it will neutralize the chemical.

Be sure to store your lye in an airtight container in a place you know children or pets cannot get into it. Also, make sure to store your soap in a safe place, as some soaps can look (and smell) tempting to pets and children.

Let's Prepare! How to Make Your Own Soap Molds

Purchasing soap molds can get expensive, and once you get the soap bug you'll likely want to spend your hard-earned money on fragrance oils and essential oils! The good news is that you don't have to spend a lot of money on soap molds. Here are a few tips for molding your soap that won't break the bank.

A great way to make round soap bars (hot process method only) is with cylindrical chip or oatmeal canisters. Clean the can out, spoon in the soap, and just tear the can off when you're ready to cut it!

I've found that yogurt containers can serve as great individual soap molds. Novelty silicone ice trays can make cute tiny soaps to pile up in a dish.

Another easy method of making your own soap molds is with milk cartons. Carefully cut the side off of a square half gallon of milk, clean it, and pour your soap in. There's no need to line the carton, as it is already lined in wax! A milk carton mold will hold approximately 2-3 pounds of soap.

If you want a bigger mold but don't want to go out and buy one, why not try a shoe box or cereal box? Be sure to line the mold with freezer paper.

Remember, you don't want your soap touching any metal besides stainless steel. Don't be afraid to get creative. Look in the baking aisle for candy molds, loaf pans, and more to shape your soap.

If you're feeling particularly crafty, why not try to make your own soap mold? I'm all thumbs when it comes to woodcraft, but if you know your way around a drill, why not try to make your own soap mold out of wood?

## Step-by-Step Cold Process Soap Making

## Overview, Pros and Cons

The term "cold" is perhaps a misnomer, as cold process soap making actually involves a bit of heat! You'll be creating this heat through chemical reactions, and you'll need to melt solid fats before mixing them. Cold process soap making is a more modern way to make soap than the hot process, but it is definitely worth it.

Cold process soap is much faster to be poured into molds than hot process soap. This cold process does involve the need for very precise mixing, but the reward is that your soap will last (make it in large quantities!). This process also requires you to wait anywhere from three to eight weeks for your soap to cure. Cold process soap making creates soap that is harder and longer lasting than the hot process method.

Step by Step How-To

Estimated time: 1.5 hours

1. Gather your Supplies

Put on your rubber gloves and goggles! Keep them on until you are completely done with all of your soap making. Make sure you have all of the supplies you need for the recipe you're using. Refer to the equipment section to see exactly what you'll be using to make your soap.

2. Prep the Lye Mixture

Carefully weigh your lye according to your recipe. To avoid spilling lye all over your scale, you can use a container or a cup (don't forget to zero the scale after putting the container) to measure your lye. Try to make the measurements as exact as possible. Measure your water into a heat resistant vessel. The recipes here will tell you exactly how much water to use, but as a general rule you should use 3 ounces of water to every 1 ounce of lye. Remember, always pour the lye into the water and not the other way around! Mix continuously until the lye is completely dissolved. Be very careful when mixing, as the chemical reaction will increase the temperature of the mixture to over 200 degrees Fahrenheit. Measure the temperature of your mixture with a thermometer and set it aside in a safe area.

3. Prep the Fatty Acids

Pour the correct weights of the oils or fats into a large pot. The measuring of these ingredients must always be done by weight for the ideal soap making results. Liquids are fine to go straight into the pot, but solid fats or oils need a little more prep. Melt your solid fatty acids in a smaller saucepan on low heat until liquid, and then add these to the large pot. Once you get more experienced making soap, you can experiment with superfatting your soap (adding extra fat) for added skin benefits of these oils. You can also add a preservative (antioxidant) to the fats and oils at this point if you so desire. Put your second thermometer in this mixture and set it aside!

4. Wait and Adjust

Most soap recipes will tell you what temperature is ideal, but generally, you want your mixtures to be between 95 and 110 degrees Fahrenheit depending on what kind of soap you're making. Make sure both of your mixtures are around the same temperature when you mix them, but it's likely that you'll have to do some adjusting. You can either put the containers in cold water or hot water.

5. Mix

Pour the lye into the fatty acids. Stir the solution constantly and rapidly. You can either use a spoon to mix in a figure eight pattern or, for much faster results, use an immersion blender. You'll know when the mixture is ready when it starts to saponify. This stage is called trace. You can test this by spooning some soap onto the surface of the liquid. If it floats, your soap is ready! If not, keep mixing. Hand mixing can take forty five minutes to an hour to reach trace, but an immersion blender can decrease this time to as little as five minutes!

6. Customize

Add the other ingredients, such as essential oils, fragrance, dyes, or exfoliants. Mix until ingredients are evenly distributed.

7. Pour into Molds and Cover

Pour the soap into your choice of mold. You can use individual molds for individual soaps, or pour your soap into a larger mold and cut it into bars after it has hardened. Cover the mold with a lid or a piece of cardboard and wrap it with lots of towels or some other fabric. The mixture is continuing to saponify while it is in the molds. It will actually get hotter before cooling off! You don't want much heat to escape, as it is essential to the early curing process. Leave the soap for anywhere to 18-36 hours (depending on the recipe).

8. Cut and Cure your Soap

If you've made your soap in a large mold, you'll want to cut it once it's solidified and is hard enough to slice. Use a sharp knife to cut your soap into even slices. If you used individual molds, gently remove the soap from the molds.

Lay your soap on a drying rack. The soap will need to cure for three to eight weeks depending on the recipe. Rotate your soap every week! When the curing process is done, make sure to wipe off any soda powder that has formed, as it can be drying on the skin. For your first few batches, you may want to test the pH level with a kit to make sure your soap is completely saponified. If your strip reads between 7 and 10, the soap is no longer caustic and is safe to touch.

9. Clean Up

It's best to wash your tools by hand to avoid leftover soap from causing your dishwasher to leak! You probably won't want to cook with your soap making pots to avoid any chemical contamination.

## Chapter 13: Tools Of The Trade

To make soap at home you'll need to invest in a few items but if you're a kitchen bug then you probably have most of what you need already. Don't worry, you can find most of what you need at affordable prices at thrift stores, dollar stores or discount retailers.

To start you'll need:

**Rubber gloves and safety goggles** - Safety comes first, my friend. To protect your eyes and hands from lye and boiling raw soap. Please don't skimp on these for they may save you an eye or a hand.

**Dish clothes or paper towels** - A rag will do as well. This is just for cleaning spills and keeping your workspace neat.

**Rubber Spatulas -** How many and how big are depending on how much soap you'll be making.

**A large spoon** - Stainless steel or plastic for mixing your lye solution.

**2/3 quart pitcher with lid** - Heat resistant plastic or stainless steel for holding your lye.

**A soap pot** - This will be for mixing your soap mixture. Pyrex pitchers are good for smaller batches (2/3 lbs) or an 8-12 quart stainless steel pot with lid for bigger batches.

**A large bowl** - for measuring your liquid oils.

**A quick reading thermometer** - for testing the temperature of your lye and liquid oils.

**A scale for measuring... everything** - Making sure your ingredients are measuring accurately is the key to making great soap.

Stainless steel measuring spoons

**Small beakers, measuring cups or ramekins** - for holding fragrance, separated soap, and colorants.

**A large ladle -** Stainless steel or plastic will do. This is to ladle out raw soap or colorants.

**A stick blender -** to blend the mixture and start the saponification process.

**A soap mold** - to pour your hot, raw soap into. You can use any leak proof container you see fit made of plastic, stainless steel or glass. You may even use wood if you line it with freezer paper first.

Finding lye may seem hard but it's actually found in most grocery stores. If you can't find one there, try a hardware store. Lye is usually found in the drain-cleaning section,

or with other products like it. If all else fails try finding an online supplier. There are dozens you can find easily and you may even be able to find essential oils or fragrances you have in mind.

Everyone has a different style to making soap. As you make your way through the basics your list of tools with grow along with your style but keep in mind you'll never go wrong with the items above.

The Fun Part!

Soap making is a frugal, creative and rewarding craft that's been around since Ancient Babylon. Whether you're an adventurous hobbyist or an aspiring business owner soap making is a wonderful investment that your skin will thank you for.

There are three main methods of making soap: the melt and pour, cold processing and re-batching. These are the easiest and most common methods for soap making for beginners. Each method will be explained with easy to follow step-by-step instructions.

Always remember to stay safe and use your safety goggle and gloves when making your soap.

The melt and pour method

This is a great method for beginners because it helps you warm up to the idea of molding your own soap with your own twist.

Step 1

Take your Pyrex pitcher and zero out the weight on your scale.

Prepare you melt and pour soap base by cutting it into small chunks then weighing enough to fit in you mold.

Quick Tip- Clear your space and soap of any dirt because it can be hard to remove once the process has begun.

Step 2

Cover the pitcher with plastic wrap with the chunks inside then place in the microwave. Set the microwave for 1 minute intervals so the soap doesn't

Every minute stir the mixture until the heat is evenly distributed. Repeat until all the chunks are dissolved.

You can also use a double broiler if you prefer.

Step 3

Zero out the weight of a ramekin then measure 4oz of any essential oil or fragrance you like. Then slowly add it to the hot soap mixture. You need to do this part slowly to prevent any bubble.

Quick Tip- If you see any bubbles try giving them a quick spray of rubbing alcohol to get rid of them.

Step 4

This next step is optional. If you want to add color to your soap then make sure to use soap safe dye or any natural colorant that won't harm your skin. Start by adding a few drops then slowly mixing to test the outcome as they can be strong. Also, feel free to blend colors if you want something unique.

Step 5

Now it's time to pour the mixture into a soap mold; be careful not to get any bubbles. The slower you pour the better the soap will take the shape of the mold.

After a few hours the soap should be set and hard enough to cut. For a quicker process you can put the molds in the refrigerator but never in the freezer. Refrigerator time should be no more than an hour.

Step 6

That was easy, right? Now all you have to do is remove the soap by tapping the back of mold. If they're hard to budge you can run warm water on the back of the mold and they should be easier to remove. Some people use a warm cloth or a knife to even out any imperfections.

Cold Processing

This is the most common method for soap makers. It's also the traditional method for making soap. Many claim that this is the best method because it results in a smoother consistency. Others say it's more versatile in what ingredients you can incorporate and when to add them. Cold Processing is the quickest way to make soap from scratch and great for beginners to try.

Step 1

Zero out the weight of your Pyrex pitcher. It's important to follow the measurements precisely when making any soap.

Prepare your oils by measuring them separately in the Pyrex pitcher then combining the solid oils in your soap pot and your liquid oils in a pitcher.

Step 2

Heat the solid oils on medium heat until it reaches 110 degrees. This is where your thermometer comes in handy. Just leave it in while it heats up so you can monitor carefully.

Now once that's at the right temperature add the liquid oils until everything reaches 100 degrees. The liquid oils will bring the temperature down as soon as you add them.

Step 3

Let the saponification begin! Dilute the lye in water and add it to the soap pot once it's ready. With the stick blender still turned off, gently stir the pot.

If you notice the oils getting cloudy, don't worry, that's supposed to happen.

Step 4

While stirring the mixture turn on your stick blender in short burst for about 3-5 seconds (continuing to stir in between). You will notice a change in the mixture as it starts to turn into soap! This is what they call trace.

Using a spoon to mix is also an option but will take you about an hour.

Step 5

The mixture will start to thicken but before it gets too thick add your fragrance and essential oils. You'll have to do this slowly, like in the melt and pour method. This is a great way to tell how your soap will smell once it's finished.

Step 6

Next add any additive to the soap like flowers, herbs or colorants. Stir these in like the fragrance without the stick blender on.

Step 7

When you feel your soap is thick enough you can pour it into your soap mold (again, very carefully). A spatula is good for getting any remaining bit in your soap pot.

Smooth out the top with your spatula and gently tap the mold on a hard surface to get rid of any air bubbles.

Unlike the melt and pour method, you have to keep the mold in a warm place and covered. The curing process needs warmth in order to saponify the right away.

Step 8

After 24 hours the soap will be hard enough to cut into whatever size you like.

Keep in mind you'll have to wait 4 weeks for your bubble bath of satisfaction. Curing may take time but it's all worth it in the end.

Re-batching

The re-batching method is typically used for soap "do over's." Instead of wasting a potentially good batch of soap you can remake it. Adjusting the fragrance, consistency and oils may need time to master but is very useful for beginners.

What to expect when re-batching:

The soap doesn't melt the same way it does in the other methods. The texture of your mixture will be a gloppy mess with a lot of clumps.

You need to put in some elbow grease if you want your re-batching to be successful. It's hard to smooth out the end result let alone tapping out the air bubbles.

If you don't know what you need to fix, chances are you won't find out while re-batching. It may be better to leave the original batch as is.

## Step 1

Minimize. Get your soap as small as you can. If the soap is hardened then using a cheese grater is a good way to get it in to tiny pieces. If it's soft, slicing it into small pieces is just fine.

## Step 2

You have a choice on what liquid you would like to melt the soap in. Plain water will do the trick but some soap makers prefer using milk because of its added benefits.

How much liquid to use depends on the age of the soap. It would be wise to start with 2-3 ounces then work your way up if you think the soap bits are not wet enough for melting.

Using too much liquid won't hurt. It will just need a longer curing process in the end.

Step 3

Recognize the issue. If the original batch didn't have enough oil you can add it once you're sure you have enough liquid for melting. If the problem was too little lye you can add it now too.

Keep in mind when adjusting lye it still needs to be mixed with water so that will also make the mixture wetter.

Step 4

Once the re-batch has melted down it will seem liquefied, almost translucent. Make sure to stir it and mash out the lumps that are still floating around.

When the liquid is wet enough to pour you can start adjusting your essential oils and other additives. Make sure they are mixed well into the soap.

Step 5

Molding will be a challenge because although it was melted the consistency of the soap will be thick and gloppy. You'll need your spatula and spoon to make sure that it smoothed into your mold. Remove the air bubbles just as you normally would.

Wait 24 hours for the re-batch to harden then try popping them out of the molds. Slice it and cure them afterwards.

Remember, the amount of time needed for curing depends on how much liquid you added to your re-batch in the initial steps.

Now that you're done with that, make a mental note on what happened or even write it down with your soap recipes. Observing your mistakes will only help improve your soap making techniques.

# Chapter 14: Basic Techniques In Making Your Soap

It is now time to decide which process of soap making you would like to use. In this chapter, you will learn how each process works and the benefits and drawbacks of each. First, there are a couple things you should know for all techniques. It is very important that you start by finding a well-ventilated area to work in. Once you find, that cover your workspace. You can use towels, a newspaper, or disposable tablecloth. The purpose of this is to protect the area and allow for safe, easy cleanup. Then you need to put on rubber gloves and safety goggles if you are going to be creating a soap that uses lye. You must also have all of your materials ready first. All of the ingredients should be exactly measured and in their appropriate containers before starting to make the soap. Make sure all the ingredients and equipment you will need in later stages is at the ready. If necessary, line your molds. It is also advisable to read your recipe thoroughly before you start. Make sure you understand the procedures you are going to be performing and the ingredients as well as the equipment you will be using. The rest of this chapter will explain to you a series of processes that can be used to make soap. The cold process, hot process, melt and pour, and rebatching techniques will be covered in-depth. Instructions for how to make liquid soap and whipped soap will also be provided.

The Cold Process

The first commonly used way of making soap is using the cold process. The advantage of the cold process is that there is a very short 'active' creation time (about 1 hour). The soap created is typically more smooth and even in texture than that produced using other procedures. Due to the fact that less lye is used in this process compared with the hot processes, this type of soap tends to be gentler on the skin. The disadvantage is that cold processed soaps need to cure for four to six weeks before using so the chemical change can complete. The first step is to create a water and lye mixture. When choosing your recipe, it will specify how much lye and how much water to combine. A good rule of thumb if your recipe does not indicate a specific amount is to use a 1-part lye, 3-part water ratio. It is very important to measure the lye by weight and preferably measure it into a container that you can close in case you need to pause or your work is interrupted. Important safety note: When combining add the lye to the water and not water to the lye for safety purposes. If the water is added to lye, there will be a chemical reaction much like putting vinegar and baking soda together. A container that can withstand high temperatures must be used for mixing because the chemical reaction between the lye and the water will cause the mixture to heat to about 200 degrees. Once the lye has been added to the water, stir continuously until the lye is dissolved or the needed reaction will not occur when you mix this combination with the oil or fat. Once combined, place a thermometer in the container and set it aside. The second step is to prepare your acid. If you are using a solid fat, melt it to liquid form. Measure your fats or oils into your soap pan using a scale. Mix the ingredients together, put a thermometer in, and set aside. Now is the time to get both of your mixtures to a temperature of around 95 degrees. This is most easily done by putting the lye container into cold water or an ice bath. You may also choose to warm your fat over the stove or in the microwave at small increments. When they are both the required similar temperature, pour the lye mixture into the fat slowly while stirring. It is important that you don't stop stirring until you reach the 'trace' phase. If you decide to hand mix, you should achieve trace in about 45 minutes. If you use a stick blender, you can reach trace in as little as 2 minutes. When using a stick mixer you do not want to turn it on and let it go to town. Instead, alternate pulses with stirring motions while the mixer is off. You know you have the right consistency, or have reached trace, when you can use your spoon to drizzle some of the substance on top of the rest and it stays there for a bit before sinking. Keep in mind that the time it takes to achieve trace can vary widely depending on temperature, stirring method, and types of fats used. Once the trace phase has been reached then fragrance, color, and anything else you wanted to add can be mixed in. Combine additives completely and pour into molds. Cover the molds with a lid and wrap in 6-8 towels. No heat should escape as it is needed for the saponification process to complete. Leave them to cure and cool for 18-36 hours. Next, remove the soap from the molds. This is the time to cut if you have decided to make bar soaps. Place the soaps on a cooling rack. Flip them every 6-8 days. The soap should be fully cured in 4-6 weeks. Surrounding the soap with open air and allowing it to harden and age as the chemical reactions stop completes this curing process.

The Hot Process

Hot process soap is more reminiscent of earlier times and of how soap would likely have been originally made. There are several advantages and disadvantages to this technique. The first advantage is that you add fragrance and color after the saponification process has occurred therefore changing their properties very little. Hot processed soap is often a bit softer making it easier to slice. On the other hand, hot processed soap is not all that easy to mold and getting a smooth top layer is difficult. Also, the process of cooking uses electricity and energy resources not required by the cold process. It is possible to use a stove, double boiler, or Crockpot to create hot processed soap. As with the cold process, you want to create your lye and water mixture in one container and your liquidized oils and fats in another pot. You do not have to wait until they reach a certain temperature to combine them when using this technique. What you want to see when mixing them together is separation. You hope to see yellowish curds on the bottom, a thick layer of oil in the middle, and white foam on the top. Once you see these layers, put the pot over low heat and stir continuously (either by hand or with mixer). If you do not stir, the solution will boil over onto the stove or counter. This is dangerous and one of the reasons you are wearing safety gear and have materials to clean up lye nearby. Cook the soap until you get bubbles that are about the size of the head of a pi. This should take about 15-25 minutes. Remove the soap from the heat and let it cool until you do not see any bubbles, about 10 minutes. Reheat on low until bubbles return. Cool again till bubbles are gone. Repeat this until no layers are left and the mixture you have is even and uniform. It should remind you of Vaseline. Add fragrance, color and any other desired additives. Pour into your molds. There is no need to insulate your molds as the saponification process has already occurred. Once the soap is cool you can remove it from molds. If needed now is the time to slice the soap. Hot processed soap can cure for as long as you feel necessary. There is discrepancy among soap makers as to whether hot process soap needs to be cured at all while some stand by curing for 4-6 weeks. It is advisable to allow at least some curing time with the soap on cooling racks.

Melt And Pour

The melt and pour technique is very popular with beginners. Using this technique is not actually soap making in the true sense because there is no saponification process. Instead, glycerin is combined with surfactants to make a soap base that can be commercially purchased. Although this process does not require the scientific prowess that other processes do, it allows the soap maker to concentrate on the aesthetics of the soap and the result can smell great and be truly beautiful. One of the major benefits of this technique is being able to avoid the use or harsh chemicals such as lye. This is particularly desirous to soap makers with children or pets who frequently enter the soap making area. Using this technique is a great way to get children involved in soap making. To make melt and pour soap, start by melting your purchased soap base. This can be done in a microwave, Crockpot, or double boiler. Then, add any additives, colors, or fragrances you wish. Now pour the soap into your mold and let it harden. Once it's hard, take it out of the mold and let it dry on cooling racks for a couple of days before using.

Rebatching

Rebatching, also called the hand milled technique, is the last process of making solid soap that we will talk about. The benefits of this process are saving money and reducing waste from not-so-pretty batches of soap. It is also a way to revive old soap that has lost its scent. Since no raw chemicals are involved, children can help make this type of soap. The first step in this technique involves making a plain soap using either the hot or cold process. Use soap to which no botanicals, dyes, or fragrances have been added. After the soap is hardened, grate it with a knife or cheese grater reserved for the purpose. Place the grated soap in a small heat proof container to microwave or put it into a mini Crockpot or a double boiler. Add nine ounces of water per twelve ounces of soap and melt it gently and gradually. It is important when using this technique to work with small batches within small containers so the soap does not burn. Do not allow the mixture to boil and be careful not to stir too much because suds and bubbles are likely to develop. Once the soap is melted, let it cool to around 150 degrees. At this point add your botanicals, fragrances, colors, etc. Now it is ready to be poured into molds. Once it is cooled, remove it from the molds. Slice if necessary and place on cooling racks for several days before storing.

Liquid Soap

Some people prefer to have liquid soap for washing hands rather than a solid bar. Liquid soap also has the benefit of being ready to use in about 3 days instead of 3 weeks. The first way to make liquid soap is to follow the recipe for a simple soap made with the cold process. Follow the instructions according to the recipe you want to use. Make sure it gets well beyond a trace before molding. Instead of curing your soap as directed, it will only sit for about three days then follow these steps:

# Conclusion

A lot of the information provided isn't just designed to help you with health and safety for yourself and your family but is also meant to be economically efficient and be better for the environment. Being conscious of health and safety extends beyond yourself and reaches into your community as well as into the world around you.

Even though the patterns and recipes in this book are deemed safe and appropriate for children, always adhere to safety precautions, especially when handling chemicals, hot items, sharp objects, and potent or concentrated items. Especially when it comes to soap making and the handling of lye.

Not only have you been provided with the plans to make your antibacterial wipes and soaps, but each chapter began with important information about the use and care of these products. If you stick to the recommendations, you will really be able to make the most out of your use of these items.

The overall purpose of this book was to provide you with plenty of material to apply to the health and safety of you and your family. The more experienced you become with working through these recipes, patterns, and plans, the more you'll be able to adapt the recipes to your specific needs. This book is meant as a starting guide for you to make DIY projects to take your health and safety into your own hands.

Remember: the items in this book are not perfect preventatives against bacteria, viruses, and germs. Nor are they curative or a substitute for medical care or professional medical advice. If you have any health concerns, it is best to consult a qualified medical professional.